Trinity College Library Dublin

This book should be returned on or before the last date shown above. It should be returned immediately if requested by the library. Fines are charged for overdue books.

Radiotherapy in practice

Radiotherapy in practice: brachytherapy
Edited by Peter J. Hoskin and Caroline Coyle

Radiotherapy in practice: external beam therapy
Edited by Peter J. Hoskin

Forthcoming volumes in the series:

Radiotherapy in practice: imaging
Edited by Peter J. Hoskin and Vicky Goh

Radiotherapy in Practice: Radioisotope Therapy

Edited by

Peter Hoskin
Professor of Clinical Oncology
University College London
and
Mount Vernon Hospital,
Rickmansworth Road,
Northwood, Middlesex
HA6 2RN

OXFORD
UNIVERSITY PRESS

OXFORD
UNIVERSITY PRESS

Great Clarendon Street, Oxford OX2 6DP

Oxford University Press is a department of the University of Oxford.
It furthers the University's objective of excellence in research, scholarship,
and education by publishing worldwide in

Oxford New York

Auckland Cape Town Dar es Salaam Hong Kong Karachi
Kuala Lumpur Madrid Melbourne Mexico City Nairobi
New Delhi Shanghai Taipei Toronto

With offices in

Argentina Austria Brazil Chile Czech Republic France Greece
Guatemala Hungary Italy Japan Poland Portugal Singapore
South Korea Switzerland Thailand Turkey Ukraine Vietnam

Oxford is a registered trade mark of Oxford University Press
in the UK and in certain other countries

Published in the United States
by Oxford University Press Inc., New York

British Library Cataloguing in Publication Data

Data available

Library of Congress Cataloging in Publication Data

Radiotherapy in practice : radioisotope therapy / edited by Peter Hoskin.
    p. ; cm. -- (Radiotherapy in practice)
  Includes bibliographical references and index.
  ISBN-13: 978-0-19-856842-1 (pbk. : alk. paper) 1. Radioisotopes--Therapeutic use.
I. Hoskin, Peter J. II. Title: Radioisotope therapy. III. Series.
  [DNLM: 1. Radioisotopes--therapeutic use. 2. Neoplasms--radiotherapy. 3. Thyroid
Diseases--radiotherapy. WN 450 R1295 2007]
  RM858.R342 2007
  615.8'424--dc22

                                                                    2006031710

ISBN 9780198568421 (Pbk.)

10 9 8 7 6 5 4 3 2 1

Typeset in Minion
by Cepha Imaging Pvt. Ltd., Bangalore, India
Printed in Great Britain
on acid-free paper by
Biddles Ltd. King's Lynn, UK

Foreword

Peter Hoskin

Unsealed radioactive sources have been used in medicine for many years for both diagnostic procedures and therapy. In current practice they are more likely to be encountered in the diagnostic setting being widely used for conventional gamma camera scanning and more recently, positron emission tomography. In contrast their use in therapy has until recently been limited, being mainly focused on treatment with radioiodine for both benign and malignant thyroid disease and occasional use of phosphorus (^{32}P) for polycythaemia and bone metastases. More recently, however, there has been a renaissance in the application of radioisotope unsealed sources in therapeutic indications. This has been stimulated by the development of chemical complexes such as the phosphonate compounds used to target bone metastasis and the neuroendocrine analogues, together with the revolution in monoclonal antibody technology, which has facilitated targeting of a radioactive isotope to sites of interest. Thus in modern medicine radioisotope therapy has an important role to play, particularly in thyroid disease, neuroendocrine tumours, bone metastasis, and non-Hodgkin lymphoma. It is an active area of research with the quest for new compounds which will be specific for therapeutic targets. Radioisotope therapy crosses many disciplines including endocrinologists, oncologists, and nuclear medicine physicians with a fundamental role for the nuclear medicine physicist in calibration, dosimetry, and administration.

Radioisotope therapy remains the nearest treatment option to the magic bullet specifically targeting sites of disease while sparing surrounding normal tissues. In many healthcare systems it may be underused where cost and lack of accessibility limit the application of radiosotopes. It is hoped this book will overcome many of these obstacles with contributions from experts in the field identifying the current role of radioisotope therapy in modern medicine and also providing a background in the physics and developmental biology that underpins their use.

Radioiodine (^{131}I) remains the most important definitive treatment for thyrotoxicosis providing targeted damage to the overactive thyroid tissue with minimal toxicity and a long established track record for safety. Similarly differentiated thyroid cancer remains unique among the solid malignant tumours in that treatment with very high doses of radiation can be delivered to provide targeted radiotherapy delivered through radioiodine administration.

The functioning neuroendocrine tumours provide a rich opportunity for radiolabelled analogues to be developed. They are taken up selectively by metabolically active tumour cells focusing radiation dose to the site of interest at a cellular level.

Bone metastases develop as a result of active osteoclastic and osteoblastic mechanisms within the bone, which result in varying degrees of remineralization. This provides opportunities for the selective uptake of phosphorous and strontium isotopes and rhenium and samarium complexes with phosphonate compounds focusing radiotherapy to sites of bone damage associated with bone metastasis. The only shortcoming of this approach is the proximity of active normal bone marrow that remains the limiting normal tissue toxicity for this treatment, which is otherwise highly effective and cost-effective. In developing healthcare systems provision of a single rhenium generator can provide sufficient isotope for multiple treatments over many months, a major impact on the substantial morbidity associated with bone metastasis.

The single greatest improvement in survival in the treatment of aggressive non-Hodgkin lymphoma has been from the introduction of monoclonal antibody drugs such as rituximab targeted against CD20. The incorporation of a radioisotope to the antibody increases efficacy further and current trials in both indolent and aggressive non-Hodgkin lymphoma are seeking to explore the potential for further increase in survival from harnessing monoclonal antibody technology with radioisotope therapy.

Barriers to radioisotope therapy relate primarily to ease of access and acquisition of radioisotopes, radiation protection regulations, and cost. Radioisotopes as an unsealed source can only be administered within a regulated environment and the risks, although small are those of spillage and environmental contamination. Many of the therapeutic radioisotopes, however, are low-energy elements, some for example strontium, having no gamma emission. As a pure beta emitter this can be given safely as an outpatient without restrictive regulations thereafter. Within a developed healthcare system access to a nuclear medicine department, oncology department, and trained physicists and physicians should not present a problem.

Contents

Contributors

Peter Hoskin
Professor of Clinical Oncology,
University College London and
Mount Vernon Hospital,
Northwood,
Middlesex, UK

Steve Evans
Head of Radiological Physics,
Royal Marsden NHS Foundation
Trust,
London, UK

Brenda Pratt
Physicist, Royal Marsden NHS
Foundation Trust,
London, UK

Barbara Pedley
Reader and Group Head: Tumour
Biology,
Department of Oncology,
Royal Free and UCL
Medical School,
London, UK

Jason Dearling
Cancer Research UK Targeting &
Imaging Group,
Department of Oncology,
Royal Free and UCL Medical School,
London, UK

Clive Harmer
Head of Thyroid Unit/Consultant in
Clinical Oncology,
Royal Marsden Hospital,
London, UK

Steve Hyer
Consultant Endocrinologist,
St Helier Hospital,
Carshalton, UK

Ujjal Mallick
Consultant Clinical Oncologist,
The Northern Centre for Cancer
Treatment,
Newcastle General Hospital
Newcastle upon Tyne, UK

Sue Clarke
Consultant in Nuclear Medicine,
Kings College Hospital,
London, UK

Jamshed B Bomanji
Consultant, Nuclear Medicine,
University College Hospital
London, UK

G Gnanasegaran
Specialist Registrar in Nuclear
Medicine,
Guy's Hospital,
London, UK

T Illidge
Professor of Clinical Oncology,
Christie Hospital,
Withington,
Manchester, UK

Yong Du
Specialist Registrar Physician,
Institute of Nuclear Medicine,
University College Hospital,
London, UK

Chapter 1

Physics principles in the clinical use of radioisotopes

Brenda Pratt, Stephen Evans

1.1 Introduction

Radionuclide therapy is a unique form of radiotherapy where the radiation dose is delivered internally to the patient. The radionuclide can be administered in a number of ways: ingestion, intravenous infusion, injection to a body cavity or pathological space, such as the cavity of a cystic glioma, or direct injection into a solid tumour. Owing to the use of 'open' or unsealed sources this type of therapy is potentially the most hazardous use of ionizing radiation in hospitals because of the potential for contamination of the environment and high external dose rates.

1.2 Physics of major radioisotopes

1.2.1 Choice of radionuclide

There are two components required for an effective therapeutic radionuclide therapy agent; first, the physical characteristics of radiation emitted by the radionuclide must provide an appropriate level of radiation dose deposition in tissue, and secondly, there needs to be a pharmaceutical or biological vector that will allow the radionuclide to be preferentially accumulated in the tumour or tissue to be treated[1,2]. The ideal therapeutic agent will provide a high localized radiation dose in the target volume, with minimal uptake in normal tissue.

When choosing a radionuclide for therapy, the physical characteristics such as the type of radiation emitted, half-life, maximum energy, and path length of the radiation need to be considered as these will all contribute to the relative biological effectiveness. Examples of the properties of common radionuclides used in unsealed source therapies are shown in Table 1.1.

1.2.2 Radiobiological considerations

The efficacy of a radionuclide therapy is dependent on the viability of the tumour cell, its relative radiosensitivity, proliferation rate, and the specificity of the radionuclide targeting. It is well known in radiotherapy that the

Table 1.1 Examples of radionuclides used in therapy[2]

Radionuclide	Half-life (T$_{1/2}$)	Emission type	Emax (MeV)
^{131}I	8.04 days	β/γ	0.6
^{90}Y	64 hours	β	2.3
^{32}P	14.3 days	β	1.7
^{153}Sm	46.3 hours	β/γ	0.8
^{89}Sr	50.5 days	β	1.5
^{186}Re	3.7 days	β/γ	1.07

Zweit J, Radionuclides and carrier molecules for therapy, Phys Med Biol 41, 1905-1914, 1996. Permission granted.

radiobiological effectiveness is greater for high-dose rate treatments than low-dose rate treatments. Radionuclide therapy is a variable dose rate treatment with the initial dose rate rapidly decreasing with time as a result of the physical decay of the radionuclide and biological clearance of the compound.

The ideal radionuclide will have a half-life that is sufficiently long to allow accumulation in the target volume and give effective treatment but not so long as to give an increased non-beneficial radiation dose[3,4].

Figure 1.1 shows the effect of (a) short half-life agent with its initial high dose rate component, and (b) a long half-life agent. In each case the shaded area shows the cumulative excess radiation dose where the dose rate is too low to compensate for cell proliferation but is still irradiating normal tissues (adapted from Dale[3]).

The biological damage caused to a cell is related to the amount of energy deposited per unit length of track and is defined as the linear energy transfer (LET). Radionuclides that provide a high LET are those that decay by emission of beta particles, alpha particles or from internal conversion (IC) or electron capture (EC). The resulting absorbed dose D, is defined as the energy imparted to matter by charged or uncharged particles and has the unit Gray (Gy) (1 J/kg =1 Gy).

1.2.3 Beta emitters

The most commonly used radionuclides in therapy are those that emit beta particles. Beta particles are emitted with a spectrum of energies and consequently have variable speeds and range. This provides a wide choice of radionuclides suitable for therapy.

The average energy of a beta particle is about one-third its maximum energy. The maximum range of a beta particle in soft tissue, in millimetres, is approximately five times its maximum energy in mega-electron volts. The range of beta particles is important in relation to the size of the tumour to be treated. High-energy beta particles are better suited to the treatment of larger

(a)

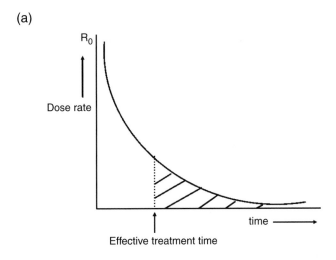

(b)

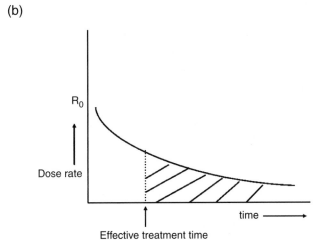

Fig. 1.1 This shows the effect of (a) short half-life agent with its initial high dose rate component and (b) a long half-life agent.[3] Reprinted from Dale RG, 'The potential for radiobiological modelling in radiotherapy treatment design', *Radiotherapy and Oncology*, **19**: 245–255, 1990, with permission from Elsevier.

volumes as in small volume disease a large fraction of the dose would be deposited in the tissues surrounding the tumour. Characteristics of some radionuclides that are beta emitters are shown in Table 1.1.

Pure beta emitters such as ^{32}P may be considered ideal as they provide a high local dose while sparing more distant tissue. Radionuclides that emit both beta and gamma radiation have an advantage of allowing uptake and distribution of the radionuclide to be imaged and or assessed; however, it also increases the radiation burden to the patient without giving any additional therapeutic benefit.

Table 1.2 β emitting radionuclides. (Δ_{np} and Δ_p are the total equilibrium dose constants for non-penetrating and penetrating radiations respectively)[5]

Radionuclide	Half-life ($T_{1/2}$) days	Average energy (MeV)	Mean range mm	Δ_{np} g Gy/ MBq/h	Δ_p g Gy/ MBq/h
^{117}Lu	6.7	0.133	0.67	0.085	0.020
^{131}I	8.0	0.182	0.91	0.109	0.219
^{153}Sm	1.9	0.229	1.2	0.156	0.035
^{186}Re	3.8	0.362	1.8	0.198	0.012
^{89}Sr	50	0.580	2.5	0.336	
^{32}P	14	0.695	2.9	0.400	
^{188}Re	0.71	0.764	3.5	0.447	0.033
^{90}Y	2.7	0.935	3.9	0.539	

Zweit J, Radionuclides and carrier molecules for therapy, Phys Med Biol 41, 1905-1914, 1996. Permission granted.

^{131}I is the most commonly used radionuclide for therapy; however, its physical properties are far from ideal. Its total equilibrium dose constant (i.e. the mean energy per unit activity and time) for penetrating radiation (Δ_p) is far higher than the respective values of the other radionuclides in clinical use (see Table 1.2). It decays with the emission of a relatively low energy beta particle, making it suitable for treating small tumours. However, two-thirds of ^{131}I decays result in penetrating medium- to high-energy gamma emissions, resulting in significant irradiation of surrounding tissues[5].

For the treatment of very small volumes or micro-metastases, short range electrons or alpha emitters would be more appropriate.

1.2.4 **Alpha particles**

Alpha particles have a maximum range of a few cell diameters (<0.1 mm) offering the possibility of cell-specific targeting with radiation of a similar range. In addition, alpha particles deposit very high LET in tissue giving an increased biological effectiveness. The potential dose from a single alpha particle is about 0.25 Gy in a 10-μm diameter cell nucleus[6]; however, owing to the very short particle range the radionuclide would have to bond to most cells within the treatment volume to be effective. Alpha-emitting radionuclides are not commonly used for radionuclide therapy because they are not readily available, are difficult to dispose of safely and have a limited clinical application. Properties of some alpha-emitting radionuclides that have been used or are considered useful for therapy are shown in Table 1.3.

Table 1.3 Properties of some α emitting radionuclides

Radionuclide	Half-life (T$_{1/2}$)	Range in tissue μm	α-particle energy (MeV)
^{211}At	7.2 hours	55	5.87
		80	7.45
^{212}Bi	60.6 minutes	57	6.05
		90	8.78
^{223}Ra	11.4 days	<100	5.78

1.2.5 Auger electrons

Radionuclides that decay by EC or IC emit low-energy characteristic X-rays and Auger electrons. These electrons have a very short range (<1 μm) and are therefore only of effective use in radionuclide therapy if the source is attached, or very close to the cell nucleus. In fact there are many radionuclides in common diagnostic use (e.g. ^{99m}Tc, ^{125}I, ^{123}I) that decay by EC but these are dispersed in the body and do not normally lead to localized high doses. There is some potential for localized administration into tumour volumes that could result in localized high-dose distributions but this is still an area of research that is outside the scope of this chapter to explore.

1.2.6 Treatment dosimetry

Traditionally treatment doses have been prescribed empirically with fixed activities given to all patients undergoing a particular treatment. The IR(ME)R regulations (see Section 9.3) require that exposures should be planned on an individual basis. Pretreatment dosimetry can be achieved using either low activities of the therapy agent such as meta-iodobenzylguanidine (m^{131}IBG) or using other isotopes of the same compound such as m^{123}IBG. In each case serial scans and external counting will provide information on the retention of the agent. The accepted method for calculating the radiation dose to tumours and whole body from radionuclide therapy has been developed by the medical internal radiation dose (MIRD) committee of the American Society of Nuclear Medicine[7]. Although MIRD may represent current best practice in this field, the doses calculated should be used with caution as they are subject to many sources of inaccuracies. For example, MIRD assumes a uniform distribution of the radionuclide within the tumour and does not distinguish between radionuclides that are bound to the cell membrane and those that are internalized within the cell or those in tissue adjacent to the tumour. It is often difficult to obtain an accurate assessment of the functioning volume of the target (tumour or organ) and details of biokinetic data for the radionuclide and the disease may be lacking.

For instance, $Na^{131}I$ and $m^{131}IBG$ are internalized within cells, which results in the beta radiation being delivered within the cell. However, with a path length of the beta radiation of the order of 0.9 mm in tissue, adjacent cells will also be irradiated.

In comparison, monoclonal antibodies are localized on cell membranes; this results in a lower ratio of tumour to normal tissue dose compared with the above radiopharmaceuticals.

1.3 Development of targeted compounds

1.3.1 Dispensing and activity measurement/validation/ QA of radiopharmaceuticals

The most common radionuclides used for therapy can be purchased from suppliers as 'ready prepared unit doses'. They will have undergone routine quality control (QC) procedures by the manufacturers and will require little in the way of further QC. However, it is always good practice to re-measure the activity prior to administration. It is usual to expect the activity available for administration to be within ±10% of the prescribed activity. A dose calibrator will give an accurate activity measurement for gamma emitters. The calibrator will have specially designed inserts to hold the most common sizes of vial and syringe in the correct measurement position. Items such as radioiodine capsules are supplied with a device to allow them to be measured in a dose calibrator. Pure beta emitters such as ^{32}P and ^{89}Sr can be more problematical as the calibration factor will change with the geometry and containment of the radionuclide. In this case the easiest method for assessing the activity is by vial subtraction. This is accomplished by measuring the stock vial activity, withdrawing the volume required for administration and then re-measuring the activity left in the stock vial.

The dose calibrator must itself be subject to regular quality assurance tests and these are described in texts such as IPEM Report 65[8].

Some radiopharmaceuticals will require further QC prior to administration; this is usually to confirm the labelling of the compound. Details of the methods of testing may be supplied by the manufacturer or can be found in text such as the *Textbook of radiopharmacy*[9] and often based around relatively simple chromatography procedures.

1.3.2 Antibodies and peptides

Tumours originate from normal cells but the process that induces malignancy results in changes on the surface of the cell such that the tumour is recognized as different from normal cells. Antibodies that recognize tumour-associated antigens can be used as a carrier of radionuclides *in-vivo* for treatment (see Chapter 2).

However, the full benefits of this type of treatment are yet to be realized. Radiolabelling of peptides has been of most therapeutic value to date, with the somatostatin analogues and in particular octreotide as the most successful (see Chapter 5). Labelling techniques are described in other texts such as the *Textbook of radiopharmacy*[9].

1.3.3 Regulatory aspects associated with radiopharmaceutical production

Radiopharmaceuticals are highly regulated being subject to regulations associated with medicinal products and ionizing radiations regulations. Their production and quality control should be managed by experienced radiopharmaceutical scientists or radiopharmacists.

Radiopharmaceuticals for research may be subject to additional regulatory restrictions and licensing. These issues are discussed further in Chapter 9.

1.3.4 Safety considerations associated with radiopharmaceutical production and administration

Preparation and dispensing of radiopharmaceuticals can result in high radiation doses to the staff involved, particularly giving high doses to the hands and fingers requiring such staff to be registered as 'classified workers'. Consideration should be given to the method and formulation of the required radionuclide. For example $Na^{131}I$ can be obtained in liquid form or as a capsule. If the dose is to be given orally then the capsule represents less of a hazard than using liquid. $m^{131}IBG$ is supplied in two formulations; one very concentrated the other dilute. The concentrated version is delivered frozen, must be thawed, dispensed, and administered within a couple of hours. The dose must be drawn from the vial(s) into a syringe, with prescribed therapy administrations of several Giga becquerals this can result in high radiation doses to the dispenser. In contrast the dilute version requires little handling by the radio-pharmacy staff and remains shielded up to the point of administration. This system is supplied with a unique giving set that allows multiple bottles to be joined together and given as a long single infusion.

References

1. Gaze MN (1991). The current status of targeted radiotherapy in clinical practice. *Physics in Medicine and Biology* **41**: 1895–903.
2. Bomanji JB, Britton KE, Clarke SEM (1995) ed. Ell PJ. 80–91 British Nuclear Medicine Society, ISBN 0 901259 11 X *Clinicians guide to nuclear medicine-oncology*.
3. Dale RG (1990). The potential for radiobiological modelling in radiotherapy treatment design. *Radiotherapy and Oncology* **19**: 245–55.

4. Dale RG (1996). Dose-rate effects in targeted radiotherapy. *Physics in Medicine and Biology* **41**: 1871–84.

5. Zweit J (1996). Radionuclides and carrier molecules for therapy. *Physics in Medicine and Biology* **41**: 1905–14.

6. Vaidyanathan G, Zalutsky MR (1996). Targeted therapy using alpha emitters. *Physics in Medicine and Biology* **41**: 1915–31.

7. Williams JR, Thwaites DI (eds) (1993). *Radiotherapy physics in practice*, pp. 289–315. Oxford University Press.

8. Gadd R, Baker M, Nijran KS, Owens S, Thomson W, Woods MJ and Zananiri F. *Protocol for Establishing and Maintaining the Calibration of Medical Radionuclide Calibrators and their Quality Control.* DTI Nutritional Measurement Good Practice Guide, 2006, ISSN 1368-6550.

9. Sampson CB (ed.) (1999). Textbook of radiopharmacy: theory and practice. Gordon and Breach Science Publishers.

Chapter 2

Antibody directed radioisotope therapy

Jason L. J. Dearling, R. Barbara Pedley

2.1 Introduction

This chapter is an introduction to the field of antibody directed radionuclide therapy. Radioimmunotherapy (RIT), brings together a number of specialities across both medicine and science. The principal components of RIT are the tumour, the antibody, and the radioisotope. The antibody, raised against antigen expressed predominantly in the tumour, acts as a vehicle delivering the toxic radionuclide. The growth and development of the tumour has important implications for the design and delivery of therapy. A greater understanding of the interaction of the antibody vector with normal tissues and with the tumour, and how this may be employed to improve efficacy, has guided efforts in antibody engineering. These factors will all be considered, along with factors influencing selection of the optimal radioisotope, which the antibody delivers to the tumour. Finally, a range of measures that can be used to maximize the effect of radionuclide therapy have been developed, and a section reporting on a representative selection of combination therapies closes this chapter. While RIT has yet to achieve its optimal efficacy in the clinic it does have great advantages over external beam radiotherapy (EBRT), including reaching small metastases deep within the body following systemic injection. Through taking advantage of improved understanding of its mechanisms of action and the strengths of RIT, its application may be of great benefit.

2.2 The target: the tumour

In the application of RIT, radiolabelled antibody (or radioimmunoconjugate, RIC) is injected into the blood as a bolus or infusion and distributes throughout the body. It is cleared from the normal tissues through metabolism and excretory pathways. Its retention is prolonged at the tumour site through its interaction with the target antigen.

2.2.1 Effect of tumour microenvironment on antibody delivery to the tumour cell

If the blood supply to the target tissue is poor then delivery of the antibody will also be hindered. Normal, non-cancerous, tissues have a strict cellular structure and an orderly, tightly controlled system of blood vessels. In healthy tissues adequate provision is made for supply of nutrients and disposal of waste products, in order that the tissue can perform its allotted task. This order does not apply to tumours. One of the characteristics of cancerous growth is a loss of control of cell behaviour and function. The cancerous cell no longer obeys the signals that guide cellular behaviour and maintain tissue structure. This leads to changes in behaviour, for example increased rate of growth, and has a number of implications. Tumour blood vessels also grow at an increased rate, and do not form and mature properly. They are spatially disorganized, tending to be more prolific at the tumour periphery, and produce a number of unusual vascular structures that affect blood flow: vessels can terminate in a blind end; fusion of vessels results in arteriovenous shunts, leading to short circuits and reversal of flow; poor formation of vessel walls can lead to their collapse. All of these reduce blood flow in the tumour, and result in vessels that might be blocked, either intermittently or permanently. This has major implications for RIT, limiting delivery and decreasing the effect of the therapy by reducing oxygen concentration in the tumour. We will consider the implications of reduced oxygen delivery in the radiobiology section of this chapter.

The antibody extravasates and moves into the tumour tissue. Molecules move out of blood vessels into surrounding tissue by diffusion and convection. Extravasation of the antibody through the endothelium into the tumour parenchyma is aided by the presence of an incomplete basement membrane and thin walls, making the vessels more 'leaky' than in healthy tissue. Poor penetration into tissue as a consequence of the large size of whole antibodies (≈150 kDa) is often a limiting factor[1] in antibody-based therapies. Movement of antibodies is governed largely by diffusion, moving down the concentration gradient. This is influenced by pressure differences within the tumour, which arise because of the heterogeneous vascular supply and its perfusion and the absent or poor lymphatic system of tumours. This gives rise to interstitial pressure that is lower at the periphery of the tumour, and then increases towards the centre, which is often necrotic. Consequently antibodies take longer to penetrate large solid tumours, limiting their efficacy as therapy vehicles.

The nature of the disease will also play a part in delivery. Large bulky tumours will be harder to access, and location might make reaching the tumour more difficult. Small metastases are likely to be the best targets for RIT, as they can be accessed, might not be detected using traditional imaging and therefore cannot be included in EBRT schedules, and a more even distribution of energy deposition can be achieved. Also higher uptake of labelled antibody has been reported in micrometastases than primary tumours in preclinical models (e.g. references 2 and 3).

2.2.2 **Antigen**

Another feature of tumour biology that will affect RIT is the nature of the target antigen. Target considerations include antigen distribution, expression levels compared with normal tissue, and accessibility. While a number of tumour-specific antigens have been identified in this review we will consider carcinoembryonic antigen (CEA) as an example, as it serves as a useful illustration of important concepts. A 180 kDa membrane-associated glycoprotein (designation CD66e), CEA was discovered in 1965[4] and is normally expressed on the apical region of cells on the luminal side of the gut, and is therefore inaccessible to intravenously injected antibody. In contrast, CEA is expressed at elevated levels on a number of common epithelial cancers, allowing for the selective targeting of antibodies. CEA is thought to have an immunological function and it is structurally capable of heterotypic and homotypic interactions, suggesting a role as a cell adhesion molecule[5]. It has been implicated in the dissemination of tumour, in particular of colorectal cancer to the liver, as it can form an interaction with a receptor on the surface of liver Kupffer cells, aiding localization of metastatic cells[6,7].

High expression of the target antigen at a concentration that ensures good localization will enable a good differential between uptake at the target site, and low residence and fast clearance from normal tissues, reducing toxicity (see Fig. 2.1). For CEA, tumour cells should express antigen in excess of 10^4 molecules per cell for effective targeting[8,9]. While an even distribution of antigen expression throughout the tumour is desirable, it is not a requirement for therapy that it be homogeneous. The radionuclides used for RIT generally have an emission range that will account for some degree of heterogeneity of antigen expression. Antigen-negative tumour cells neighbouring antigen expressors will still be included in the therapy in what is termed cross-fire, or the bystander effect[10,11].

If the antigen is shed from the tumour cells into the blood this might lead to faster clearance of the antibody from the blood. High serum CEA concentration (e.g. >1000 µg/l) bar a patient from receiving RIT in clinical trials. Complexes of antigen and antibody in the blood are cleared via the liver, reducing targeting efficiency, though given the usually low amounts of antigen in blood this is of more importance to imaging than therapy. The amount of CEA in the serum

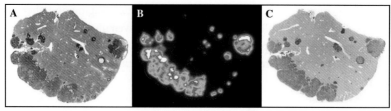

Fig. 2.1 Tumour localization of radiolabelled antibody. This image demonstrates the strength of RIT—the radioactivity localizes to the tumour site and clears from the normal tissues. These are sections from a preclinical model of intrahepatic colorectal cancer metastases. The first image (A) is a tissue section that has been stained using haematoxylin and eosin to demonstrate the liver (light pink) and tumour (dark purple) (scale bar = 2 mm). Radiolabelled antibody ([^{125}I]A5B7, a whole IgG raised against carcinoembryonic antigen, CEA) was administered intravenously 48 hours before the tissue was taken. The position of the radionuclide within the tissue was detected before staining using quantitative autoradiography (B is a digital image of the autoradiograph). Tissue uptake was calculated to be 14.54 % injected dose per gram (%ID/g) in tumour and 0.327 %ID/g in liver, a tumour to normal ratio of 44.4:1. The specificity of localization to the tumour cell is dependent on its predominant expression of antigen compared with normal tissue. Expression of CEA has been demonstrated in C using immunohistochemistry—brown staining indicates antigen binding by A5B7, detected using an immunoperoxidase reaction producing a brown stain, while tissue without antigen counterstains blue with haematoxylin.

might be used as a guide to tumour volume, though there are conflicting data on this from preclinical models[12,13]. Differences in serum content of antigen between models of primary and metastatic disease have been reported[2,3]. While the relationship between serum CEA and faster clearance of the RIC from the blood has been described there is also evidence that the type of tumour and site of metastasis are also influential[14].

Having discussed the target site and some of the challenges faced by RIT we now consider the vehicle to be used, and how developments in molecular biology and protein engineering have increased our understanding of the mechanisms at play.

2.3 Antibodies as vehicles for radiotherapy

Antibodies are glycoproteins produced by B lymphocytes and form the soluble receptor of the B-cell recognition of antigen. They are bi-functional molecules comprising an antigen-binding moiety and an immunological effector moiety, forming an integral part of the immune defence system. Antibody subclasses and molecular structures have been described extensively elsewhere.

An ideal targeting antibody would be cleared from normal tissues but retained in tumour tissue through association with membrane-associated molecules, against which the antibodies were raised and are uniquely or overly expressed by some or all of the target cells. While Ehrlich described antibodies as 'magic bullets' in 1913, making reference to their specificity, it was not until 1975 that the development of hybridoma technology[15] allowed the production of monoclonal antibodies (mAb) possible for widespread investigation and use.

A targeting antibody is cleared from normal tissues but retained in tumour tissue through association with membrane-associated molecules against which the antibodies are raised, and are uniquely or overly expressed by some or all of the target cells.

As a therapy targeting molecule the most widely used class is IgG, with long residence time in the circulation enabling good tumour localization. However, prolonged serum persistence of an IgG-based RIC can result in bone marrow toxicity as well as increase the likelihood of an immune response from the host. To overcome these potential limitations, antibodies properties such as size, affinity, avidity, and immunogenicity have been engineered in order to produce more optimal targeting molecules.

2.3.1 Antibody engineering

Initially rodent antibodies, generally mouse, were used in research, though rat antibodies have the advantage of higher stability and higher productivity of producer cells[16]. Advances in antibody engineering have now been made possible by developments in molecular biology. The use of display technologies to select the appropriate protein, which reacts with the target antigen but not normal tissues, and expression systems to produce these in large quantities, have contributed to the rapid developments in this field.

Display technologies include phage systems, *in vitro* display on ribosomes, and cell surface systems displaying antibody fragments on the surface of bacterial or yeast cells. They all have the common property of the display format—recovery of both the mature protein and the genetic information by physically linking the genotype to the phenotype[17,18]. This property offers a powerful means of rapidly screening large antibody libraries to select for the desired antibody characteristic (e.g. antigen specificity, affinity, stability).

Systems employed in the large-scale production of antibody proteins include both eukaryotic and prokaryotic cells. Mammalian cell lines including hybridoma and recombinant CHO cell lines[19,20], insect cells and plants[21,22] have been described. Required properties of an ideal systems are high titre, low cost, and swift production times. Consequently, bacteria and yeast expression systems are most commonly used. These can vary in protein processing, folding, and post-translational modifications.

Size

Figure 2.2 shows a range of antibody formats commonly employed in clinical trials. Larger antibody molecules will generally have higher absolute localization in the tumour, mainly because of long circulation time, but poorer penetration into the tissue. Smaller molecules have greater potential for penetration into the tumour tissue, but will clear more quickly from the blood, predominantly through the kidney, achieving higher tumour to normal tissue ratios, but at the cost of absolute uptake. Protein engineering has gradually reduced the size of the antibody down to the smallest constitutive part that recognizes antigen in order to produce targeting molecules that will combine high tumour uptake with high tumour to normal tissue ratios.

Commonly used recombinant antibody fragments are Fabs—these consist of the V_L–C_L and V_H–C_{H1} chains, which are linked by disulphide bonds (Mw ≈55 kDa). However, the presence of two chains can complicate genetic manipulation and large-scale production of these molecules. The rapid clearance and monovalent nature of Fab fragments means that they have been more successful in larger, multivalent formats[23–29]. For example, it has been shown in a comparative clinical study that F(ab′)2 fragments localize more rapidly to the tumour than the parent IgI[30] giving higher maximal dose rates.

The most widely used combination of V_H and V_L domains is the single chain Fv antibody fragment (scFv, MW of ≈27 kDa). In this form the V_H and V_L

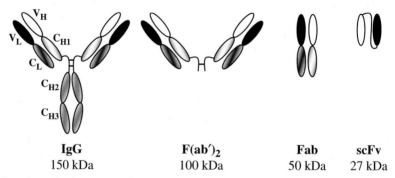

| **IgG** | **F(ab′)$_2$** | **Fab** | **scFv** |
| 150 kDa | 100 kDa | 50 kDa | 27 kDa |

Fig. 2.2 Antibody construct formats. This schematic shows the range of antibody formats made available through advances in molecular biology. Larger molecules give higher absolute tumour uptake, but have poorer tumour penetration and longer blood pool residence time leading to greater toxicity. Smaller molecules clear from the blood more quickly, but at the cost of lower absolute tumour localization. Therefore, smaller molecules tend to be used for imaging and larger molecules for therapy.

domains, which otherwise dissociate and aggregate, are tethered using a flexible linker[31,32]. These small molecules exhibit rapid clearance from blood, monovalent binding to antigen and low accumulation in the tumour with high kidney uptake[33–40]. Incorporation of scFv as building blocks in larger molecules, including their fusion to enzymes[41,42], cytokines[43], and albumin (44) or into multivalent formats (see Avidity section below) has resulted in improved pharmacokinetics.

Affinity

One of the most important performance criteria for antibodies is the strength of binding (affinity) to the antigen—without this property the antibody will not localize to the tumour. Affinity can be defined by the equilibrium binding constant of the antibody/target antigen interaction. The dissociation constant K_D is equal to k_{off}/k_{on} where k_{on} is the association of the antibody on to the antigen and k_{off} is the dissociation of the antibody off the antigen.

Antigen binding occurs through non-covalent bonds formed between amino acids on the topological surface of the antigen and the antibody binding site. Improvements to the antibody/antigen interaction can be engineered into the antibody binding site using structural knowledge, antibody display approaches or a combination of both. There has been conflicting evidence of this *in vivo*—increasing affinity has been shown to have either a beneficial[45–49] or no effect[50] on tumour localization. While it is certainly important for the antibody to have a high affinity, there may be a threshold above which increase in affinity results in no further tumour localization and other factors become limiting[8]. High affinity might hinder tumour penetration by the antibody—the binding site barrier[51,52] reduces antibody uptake by inhibiting movement into the tumour following binding of extravasated antibody to the nearest accessible antigen. This effect is particularly significant when large amounts of protein are administered.

Avidity

Having more than one potential antigen binding region on the antibody is referred to as multivalency. Increasing the avidity of an antibody produces an overall increase in binding. The affinity effect is amplified and the antibody molecule has an increased functional affinity or avidity[53]. IgG have two antigen-binding regions and so bind antigen with functional affinity. To improve the tumour retention of monovalent scFv and Fab antibody fragments they have been engineered into multimeric constructs using a variety of chemical and genetic cross-linkages. Methods to increase the avidity of svFv include cross-linking two scFv molecules by incorporating a free cysteine residue into the sequence and this method of increasing avidity has been shown to increase tumour localization[37,54]. A simpler method is to link two scFv molecules into a single polypeptide, which can also improve tumour localization[55]. Another successful method to increase the avidity of scFv molecules is based on the non-covalent association of the VH chain of one scFv with the VL chain of another[56]. Preclinical studies using divalent formats (diabodies) have demonstrated high functional affinity, greater tumour retention, and slower systemic clearance than their monovalent counterparts[57].

Immunogenicity

Systemic administration of murine mAbs can lead to immune responses in the form of human antimouse antibodies (HAMA) usually directed against the Fc regions of the immunoglobin[57]. An immune response will lead to faster clearance of the antibody through the development of immune complexes and preclude repeat treatments. This has led to the development of chimeric, humanized, and fully human antibodies in an effort to reduce interspecies differences.

Chimeric antibodies combine the Fab fragment of a murine antibody with a human Fc region. The antibody can be further humanized by transferring just the CDR loops on to a human framework. Fully human antibodies are produced using transgenic mice with human immunoglobulin genes[58–60]. Fully human scFv and Fab antibody fragments may also be isolated from human antibody libraries on the surface of phage[61]. Recombinant antibodies can also be 'resurfaced' to present a more human Fv framework[62,63].

Unconjugated 'naked' antibodies normally exert their effect through apoptosis initiation, interference with ligand–receptor interactions, the anti-idiotype network, complement-mediated cytotoxicity or antibody-dependent cell-mediated cytotoxicity. While the properties of the antibody will influence the outcome of RIT, it is primarily the characteristics and emissions of the nuclide that will result in a therapeutic effect. We will now consider the properties of different nuclides that can be used in RIT, factors affecting isotope selection, and the effects of targeted radiotherapy on the tumour.

2.4 Selection of radioisotope and its effect on the tumour

The choice of radioisotope for use in RIT is guided by availability, ease of use, cost, and effects on both the tumour and normal tissues. The bombardment of suitable parent atoms with particles, such as neutrons or helium particles, in a nuclear reactor or accelerator produces unstable radioisotopes. These have chemical properties identical to their stable equivalents, but will have physical decay properties defined by their nuclear characteristics. Emissions produced vary according to the decay of the radioisotope, and the biological effect will vary with the emission. A well-defined and described chemistry will aid in the use of the isotope. The half-life of the nuclide should be amenable to purification, transport from site of production to place of use, and radiopharmaceutical production. Provision of the radioisotope should be at a suitable specific activity and in an amenable form for use in a clinical setting.

Therapeutic radioisotopes achieve their toxic cellular effects through the interactions of their emissions with cellular components, in particular the DNA. There are three types of emission employed in RIT—Auger electrons, α and β^- (see Table 2.1).

Auger electrons

These are high-energy emissions that are very toxic, but their short path length ($\approx$0.1–5 μm) means that they have optimal effect when attached to an internalizing antibody. The relative biological effectiveness (RBE, a measure of the biological activity of an emission as compared with a standard) of an Auger-emitting radioisotope is increased greatly by cellular internalization[64]. The most widely investigated examples of Auger emitting radioisotopes are ^{111}In and ^{125}I.

α particles

Alpha particles are essentially helium nuclei, that is two neutrons and two protons. As these have a large mass they can prove very toxic compared with β^- emissions (see reference 65), especially if introduced into the cell. Radioisotopes that emit α particles often require generation in a reactor, specialist handling and chemical techniques, and are also short-lived, giving little opportunity for antibody labelling or localization to the tumour site. Studies using these isotopes have therefore been largely limited to proof of principle preclinical studies and those using locally introduced RIT for treatment of organ surface tumours (e.g. see references 66 and 67). Despite the difficulties involved in the use of these isotopes their toxicity makes them attractive for future studies. Given rapid accumulation at the tumour site and the potentially devastating nature of their emissions there is also interest in use of these nuclides in vascular targeting[68,69].

β^- emissions

These are electrons which travel further through tissue than either Auger or α emissions, but are not as toxic. So for example, the E_{max} for the ^{131}I β^- decay is 610 keV, and this loses 90% of its energy at 0.83 mm from the site of disintegration, while the E_{max} for ^{90}Y the β^- decay is 2270 keV and 90% of its intensity is lost at 5.2 mm[70].

Table 2.1 Radioisotopes suitable for use in radioimmunotherapy. Imaging radionuclides are given where they are either widely used for radioimmuno detection of cancer (e.g. ^{99m}Tc), or if their physicochemical properties suggest them as scouting radionuclides appropriate for use in conjunction with a therapeutic nuclide (producing a 'matched pair'). Only the most relevant emission is given. Some nuclides are more versatile, having both therapeutic and imaging emissions. An example is ^{64}Cu, β^- 39%, 0.578 MeV (therapeutic—the disintegration of ^{64}Cu also produces some Auger emissions) and β^+ 19% 0.65, and EC 41%, both of which can be used for imaging

Radioisotopes	Emission energy (MeV)	Physical $T_{1/2}$
Imaging		
γ		
^{99m}Tc	0.142	6.01 h
^{111}In	0.173, 0.247	2.805 days
β^+		
^{64}Cu	1.675	12.701 h
^{89}Zr	0.9	3.27 days
^{124}I	1.53	4.18 days
Therapy		
Auger		
^{111}In	0.86	2.805 days
^{123}I	1.234	13.2 h
^{125}I	0.179	60.1 days
α		
^{149}Tb	3.97	4.13 h
^{211}At	5.980	7.21 h
^{212}Bi	6.051	1.009 h
^{213}Bi	8.537	0.8 h
^{223}Ra	5.3–5.9	11.435 days
^{225}Ac	5.3–5.8	10 days
β^-		
^{67}Cu	0.58	2.58 days
^{90}Y	2.282	2.67 days
^{131}I	0.606	8.04 days
^{177}Lu	0.497	6.75 days
^{186}Re	0.973	3.78 days
^{188}Re	2.118	16.94 h
^{199}Au	0.292	3.14 days

Radioisotopes with β^- emissions are currently the most widely used in targeted radiotherapy. Those with short emissions deliver the absorbed dose to the tumour site, restricting toxicity to tumour rather than surrounding, normal tissue. This is particularly important in the treatment of micrometastases. Isotopes with a longer range will spread their delivered dose over a wider range, and reduce the heterogeneity of dose. Therefore, more energetic emissions might be better for larger tumour deposits (e.g. reference 71). As well as providing an advantage by the cross-fire effect, regions of tumour, which might not be reached by the RIC itself, will be affected by radionuclide emissions. It has been suggested that a mixture of radioisotopes might prove an advantage for therapy[72]. The energy of an emission is deposited in tissue at a certain rate along the length of the track travelled, and this is referred to as the linear energy transfer rate (LET, units keV/μm) of the emission. An emission with a high LET (e.g. an α particle) will cause more damage per unit length, and therefore be more toxic than a low LET emission (e.g. a β emission). However, a high LET particle will not travel very far, so a more homogeneous distribution throughout the tumour is required for a successful therapy.

The half-life of the radioisotope should be about 1.5–3.0 times that of the peak uptake time in the tumour. Mathematical modelling has investigated the relative merits of longer and shorter nuclide half-lives, with indications that longer-lived radioisotopes may have some advantage[71,73].

Currently the most widely used radioisotopes in RIT are ^{131}I and to a lesser extent ^{90}Y. This is due to a combination of properties including: ease of production; a half-life amenable to transport, RIC preparation and localization to the tumour; a medium energy of β⁻ emission, limiting energy deposition primarily to the tumour; and, in the case of ^{131}I, imageable γ emissions. The high-energy γ emissions of ^{131}I (900 keV) increase dose to the patient's normal tissues and to staff, while the relatively long half-life makes disposal of clinical waste problematic. This confers a relative advantage on ^{90}Y, but this is lessened by the more complicated labelling procedure requiring use of a chelator, and the potential for radiotoxicity to normal tissues both from the long emission range of the isotope, and from the redistribution of ^{90}Y to the skeleton following catabolism of the RIC.

2.4.1 Antibody radiolabelling

There are two methods for the attachment of the nuclide to the antibody vehicle—direct and indirect techniques. Direct radioiodination is the reaction of iodine with ring structures, such as the phenol ring of tyrosine, on the antibody surface, in the presence of an oxidizing agent, such as chloramine-T[74] or IODO-GEN (tetrachlorodiphenylglycouril). Briefly, the antibody is suspended in buffer at a concentration of not normally less than 1 mg/ml, and the radioiodine is added. This is followed by addition of, for example, chloramine-T, then after a brief exposure L-tyrosine to quench the reaction. The mixture now contains labelled protein and non-protein-associated iodine, which are separated by use of a desalting column. The labelled protein is eluted from the column before the rest of the 'free' iodine. Radiopharmaceutical purity is assessed by thin-layer chromatography (e.g. stationary phase silica gel, mobile phase 80%:20% methanol/water), and antigen binding by use of an affinity column bearing the target antigen. These general directions vary for the protein and for the desired product. For example, if the protein is known to be susceptible to oxidation damage then IODO-GEN-coated beads or tubes can be used instead of chloramine-T, though this requires a longer exposure time (e.g. 1 minute for chloramine-T and 20 minutes for IODO-GEN). Antioxidants (such as ascorbic acid) might be used to end the reaction and in the storage of the RIC. While this generic method is suitable for ^{125}I and ^{131}I, use of the positron-emitting [124]I has been hindered due to technical difficulties, though recent advances will aid its use[75].

Increasing the number of iodine molecules on the antibody can interfere with the interaction with antigen, potentially decreasing tumour localization. This can be due to iodine in the binding site. Direct labelling is subject to enzymatic breakdown *in vivo*, as the products can be prone to endogenous iodases, and internalized antibodies might be metabolized by lysosomal degradation to monoiodotyrosine. Both of these routes of degradation could contribute to a decreased tumour residence time of the radionuclide and therefore a decrease in efficacy of the therapy. Indirect, and more stable, methods of attaching iodine to proteins have been developed such as *N*-succinimidyl *para*-hydroxyphenylpropionate[76], which can be used in much milder conditions (see references 77 and 78 for further examples). Reducing the amount of free iodine or iodotyrosine in this way leads to significant changes in the biodistribution of antibodies, including changing the amounts of activity found in the stomach and neck/thyroid[54,79]. Tumour uptake was found to increase substantially when a 'residualizing' iodine label was used, compared with chloramine-T labelling[80]. This label is retained lysosomally following catabolism, and increased predicted dose to the tumours by eightfold compared with conventionally labelled antibody.

The indirect method of labelling the protein uses a bifunctional chelator, a chemical linker, which attaches the protein to the radionuclide. These are also available for use with metallic radionuclides such as ^{111}In and [90]Y. Diethylenetriaminepenta acetic acid (DTPA) can be used as a chelating molecule with indium though for other metals, such as yttrium, DOTA (1,4,7, 10-tetraazacyclododecane—*N,N',N'',N'''* tetraacetic acid) metal complexes have higher stability.

2.4.2 **Radiolabelled antibody distribution**

Knowledge of the pharmacokinetics of the radiolabelled antibody in the body and its distribution within the tumour, coupled with an appropriate choice of radioisotope, are critical steps in achieving optimal therapy.

The antibody is injected into the blood and circulates through the body, being retained in the tumour by its interaction with the target antigen. The amount of radioactivity in the tumour increases until a peak is reached and then decreases because of both the biological half-life of the antibody and the physical half-life of the radioisotope. The extent and duration of uptake, both critical factors in determining the total absorbed dose and probability of tumour control, are influenced by: clearance of the radiolabelled antibody from blood, which limits the amount available to localize to the tumour; accessibility of the tumour; properties of the antibody; stability of the labelling; and the membrane half-life of the target antigen.

It has been reported that an inverse relationship exists between the size of the tumour and the dose delivered from RIT in preclinical and clinical studies[50,81,82] and that higher dose rates in smaller tumours lead to better chances of successful therapy[83]. This might suggest that the best target for RIT is disseminated disease comprised of micrometastases throughout the body, untreatable by either EBRT or surgery. Furthermore, it is difficult to detect micrometastatic deposits using current medical imaging techniques (imaging resolution of 0.5 cm at best). Therefore RIT could be employed in an adjuvant or prophylactic role, delivering therapy to as yet undetected metastatic deposits, following conventional therapies.

Pretargeting dosimetry can be used to design an optimal therapy on an individual basis. Radiolabelled antibody is given to the patient and then imaging (e.g. single photon emission computed tomography/positron emission tomography, PET) throughout a time course is used to identify those patients in whom the antibody localizes to the tumour, and eliminate those who would not be effectively treated by RIT. The optimal amount of radiolabelled antibody for greatest effect on the tumour, given acceptable toxicity, can then be calculated. A small amount of therapeutic nuclide, which also has imageable emissions, such as ^{131}I or ^{186}Re can be used for this. It is more acceptable to administer an isotope with imageable emissions for which there is an isotope of the same element with therapeutic emissions, such as ^{90}Y (β^-) and ^{86}Y or ^{89}Zr (PET)[84]. Other 'matched pairs' are ^{99m}Tc (γ) and ^{188}Re (β^-), or ^{124}I (PET) and ^{131}I (β^-). The problem with this approach is that: it involves administration of radioactivity to patients in addition to the therapeutic treatment, and might exclude some of them from further treatment; there is an inhomogeneous dose distribution at a much smaller scale than can be imaged within the tumour, leading to a wide dose variability; prediction of outcome is very difficult. Some work has been carried out to systematically match the radionuclide and antibody on the basis of clearance, half-life, and track length of emission[72,85] so that the efficiency of an imaging or therapy system can be optimized.

2.4.3 Radiobiology: the interaction of radionuclide emissions with cells

Having chosen the molecule and radionuclide and delivered it to the tumour site, the effect that this will have on the tumour and its constituent cells must be considered. There are a number of similarities and differences in the application and mechanisms of action of the more mainstream EBRT and the emergent therapy RIT. Discussion of these illustrates the relative strengths and weaknesses of each modality.

There is a relationship between the dose delivered (D) and the surviving fraction of cells (S_f), i.e. their radiosensitivity. The resulting graph will be linear (given a logarithmic y-axis) for high LET radiation. For lower LET radiation a shoulder appears at low doses, caused by repair of sublethal damage (SLD), but the linear response is still seen at higher doses. This relationship between the surviving fraction of cells (S_f) following an instantaneous dose (D) may be described using the linear quadratic formula[86].

$$S_f = e^{-(\alpha.D + \beta.D2)}$$

where α and β do not refer to the type of radiation but give an indication of the radiosensitivity of the tissue, relating to cellular damage arising from single (α) or multiple (β) track events. The a term is of primary importance, and should be in the range 0.35–0.5 Gy^{-1} for radiocurative tumours. The α/β ratio gives an indication of whether a tissue is likely to be late or early responding[86,87]. For example, late responding tissues will have an α/β ratio of about 3–4, while early responding tissues will be in the larger range of 5–20[86]. The response curve for RIT might be higher than for EBRT, i.e. a poorer response might be expected from RIT than for EBRT, contributed to by the mechanisms outlined below[88]. The inherent radiosensitivity of tissues varies, with lymphomas responding to ≈15 Gy and colorectal carcinomas requiring more than four times as much radiation for a therapeutic effect[89].

The effect of periodic EBRT irradiation on the tumour is often considered conceptually in terms of the stripping away of layers of onion skin. The outer, better perfused, normoxic region of the tumour is more susceptible to irradiation and therefore bears the brunt of the therapy. Through a combination of tissue remodelling and decrease in the metabolic consumption of oxygen the previously hypoxic regions are reoxygenated before they are consequently irradiated.

The therapy time of RIT allows for the reoxygenation of hypoxic regions, which are inherently more resistant to radiation, but this is not seen in all tissue types. There is evidence that the response of tumours to RIT is more complex, with variations in timing and extent of reoxygenation both between and within tissue types (reference 90 and references therein).

The antibody localization, and therefore region of irradiation, in the body is not limited to a discrete, defined region as in EBRT, but rather will localize in any region of the body that is involved in disease and is accessible via the blood stream. Medical imaging directs field arrangements for EBRT, but in their interpretation regions of tumour might be missed. Therefore, RIT has the advantage that it will also target outlying regions of tumour at the primary site not identified by imaging or surgery and micrometastases distant from the identified primary cancer site.

EBRT has a defined time schedule while RIT does not. The radiolabelled antibody builds up in the tumour and starts to have an effect on the cancer cells. Therapy effectively begins when sufficient toxicity is being delivered to overcome the number of cells being produced by proliferation, i.e. when there is a negative net effect on tumour cell number (at dose rate R_{crit}). The therapy ends when R_{crit} is again reached (at time T_{crit}). This period, for a whole IgG combined with ^{131}I, is typically around a week.

Through careful use of a well-planned field arrangement a homogeneous distribution of dose throughout the identified tumour volume is possible in the application of EBRT. However, the dose is delivered heterogeneously to the tumour in RIT due to a combination of delivery, heterogeneity of antigen expression throughout the tumour, and the path length of the emission. The radioisotope localizes initially to the outer, growing front of the tumour, which may contribute to the greater effect per unit of absorbed dose for RIT compared with EBRT[91]. The total tumour dose delivered by RIT is also lower than for EBRT, though positive therapy outcomes have been reported. A number of studies comparing the efficacy of RIT and EBRT have been undertaken[92–95]—for overview see reference 91). These have mainly involved the use of preclinical models and either the direct detection of dose delivered to the tumour using implanted thermoluminescent detectors (TLDs) or its calculation using methods involving autoradiography. A range of different models, antibodies, and nuclides have been investigated, making direct comparisons difficult.

It is considered that the principal site of radiation damage of the cell is the DNA. This could be damaged in two ways: either by a single hit causing irreparable damage, such as a double strand break, or through two coincidental interactions, such as two single strand breaks causing cell death. External beam therapy is given at a high dose rate (e.g. 360 cGy/min) for a brief period (e.g. usually for a total of 2 Gy). In RIT the dose is given at a very low-dose rate for an extended period. During RIT it is possible that a cell might suffer a single strand break, which could then be repaired before another single strand break occurs—the probability of this happening depends on both the dose rate and the rate of repair. The repair of sublethal, or potentially lethal, damage before it is promoted to lethal damage is therefore more relevant to the success of RIT than EBRT, and may require a 20% increase in dose to overcome. However, low-dose rates (about 5–300 cGy/h)[96] can hinder cell proliferation, imposing a partial G_2/M block, though cells can still progress through the cycle. This will lead to a synchronization of cells in the G_2 phase, which is more radiosensitive, suggesting an advantage for low-dose rate RIT over EBRT.

Cells that have a low concentration of oxygen or are hypoxic, due to their distance from perfused vessels, are termed chronically hypoxic, and those that are rendered hypoxic for short periods, often due to vascular occlusion, are acutely hypoxic. All tumours examined to date, from both preclinical and clinical sources, contain areas of hypoxia, even in the case of micrometastases (<1.0 mm diameter). Changes in cellular metabolism render chronically hypoxic cells resistant to a range of non-irradiative cancer therapies[97].

Hypoxic cells are also significantly more radioresistant to RIT than normoxic cells. Oxygen plays an important part in the death of a cell following irradiation. The emissions from the radioisotope deposit energy in the cell, causing damage either through direct or indirect means. Alpha particles (essentially a helium nucleus), will directly affect the structure of important molecules, such as DNA. Less energetic emissions, such as β^- particles, rely more for their toxic effect on indirect effects. As the particle traverses the cell free radicals are created, mostly involving oxygen (such as superoxide O_2^-, and hyperoxide $H_2O_2^-$). These then interact with, among other molecules, cellular DNA to cause damage and lead to cell death. Acute hypoxia typically lasts for short periods of time[98], and therefore probably does not impinge on RIT given the relatively long period of radiolabelled antibody retention in the tumour, but is more of a concern for EBRT. The difference between the radiation dose required for a cytotoxic effect and the dose required under hypoxia for the same effect is termed the oxygen enhancement ratio (OER). The OER for high-dose rate radiotherapy is about 2.5–3.0. The OER at lower doses[99–101] and lower dose rates[102–104] is lower. That is, hypoxic cells are not as resistant to low-dose rate therapy, such as RIT, as they are to high-dose rate therapy. Whereas a high-dose rate OER might be of the order of 2.5 to 3, the OER for a low-dose rate therapy might be of the order of 1.3–2, the variations due to differences in cell line response and the RBE of the nuclide. However, it has been shown that better oxygenated tumours demonstrate a greater response to RIT[105], and that administration of an agent that increases the oxygen carrying capacity of the blood (a perfluorocarbon) increases the reponse of tumours to EBRT at a rate comparable with that delivered by RIT[106]. The OER for RIT will also depend on the LET of the radioisotope—higher LETs produce a lower OER. The reason for this sensitization of hypoxic cells to low-dose rate therapy is the effect of prolonged low oxygen concentration on repair mechanisms, which are compromised by the metabolic changes that occur as a consequence of long-term hypoxia.

Experiments carried out to measure this effect are dogged by technical difficulties. It requires a period of time to deliver a measurably cytotoxic dose to cells at a low-dose rate. Cells under low concentrations of oxygen die, confounding analysis of data. Plastic and glassware can retain an oxygen reservoir. The extent of this, and its implications for experiments requiring low oxygen levels, was not appreciated until the early 1970s. Oxygen depletion due to radiolysis and metabolic usage can alter oxygenation. Recreating the *in vivo* environment *in vitro* is also problematic, and can render translating data to the clinic difficult.

The biological, temporal, and physical factors affecting RIT are complex and interrelated. RIT might be enhanced, or be complemented by other therapy modalities. Analysis of the outcome of these combinations provides further insight into mechanisms of action, as well as ways of employing RIT gainfully in the clinic.

2.5 Improving the efficacy of radioimmunotherapy

Various ways of improving RIT have been considered, based on understanding its mechanism of action, and its limitations. The three components, the tumour, the antibody, and the radioisotope, must be considered. A representative selection are discussed below.

2.5.1 Increasing tumour uptake of the radioimmunoconjugate

Methods of maximizing the effect of the administered RIC and increasing tumour uptake take account of: location and type of tumour; maximum dose that can be administered, limited by normal tissue toxicity; and the need for the antibody to extravasate and interact with the target antigen.

As noted earlier the site and nature of the tumour can influence the success of therapy. Tumours that are sited on the surface of organs, or that are intraperitoneal, may be better accessed using local injection. This technique could also make use of short half-life isotopes, such as α-emitters, more feasible, reducing toxic effects and increasing localization at the tumour site. Refinements in the more appropriate use of radiation, including patient selection and use of the correct radioisotope, have been suggested. Clinical use of RIT for solid tumours has yet to become widespread, but the use of RIT for adjuvant therapy, or as a prophylactic measure where metastases could cause future disease, have been suggested[107]. Similarly appropriate use of radioisotopes extends to matching the characteristics of the radioisotope to the antibody and to the tumour for maximum effect.

The principal dose-limiting tissue in RIT is usually the bone marrow. The radio-labelled antibody is initially injected into the patient's blood, and therefore has access to the marrow, which is a relatively radiosensitive tissue ($\alpha/\beta = 2.5$ Gy, $\alpha = 1.5$ Gy^{-1}, $\beta = 0.6$ Gy^{-2})[108]. For dosimetry purposes it is assumed that 36% of the radioactivity in the blood is in the bone marrow[109]. This dose-limiting effect can be overcome in a number of ways, including by bone marrow transplantation rescue[110,111], by increasing the radioresistance of the bone marrow through the use of colony-stimulating factors[112,113], or by fractionating the dose. Dose fractionation means that rather than giving a single injection of radiolabelled antibody the dose is split into smaller injections given over a period of time. Radiolabelled antibody clears from normal tissues allowing them to repair during the later phase of each therapy. In contrast, tumour tissue retains the radioactivity longer than the normal tissues, receiving a relatively constant low-dose rate depending on the spacing of individual treatments. By reducing the toxicity to the normal tissues in this way, a greater total amount of activity could be administered—for example, 15–20% more for the same bone marrow toxicity as measured by granulocyte and platelet levels[114]. Studies into a variety of regimens based around fractionated RIT have found both against[115] and in favour of fractionation, where lower normal tissue toxicity has been reported for a similar, if not improved, tumour response, in terms of survival and tumour regression[116–119]. Variations are probably due to the interval between doses and tumour growth characteristics. Caveats for this approach include reduced tumour uptake of serial injections of antibody, possibly due to vessel damage and reduced target tumour mass due to the action of the therapy[120].

EBRT irradiation of the tumour site in combination with RIT increases the tumour response by combining the two therapies at the tumour site as well as causing vascular damage, increasing tumour uptake of antibody. However, use of EBRT requires knowledge of the site and extent of disease, and cannot be used throughout the body in the therapy of micrometastases.

Hyperthermia, heating the tumour, has been found to increase the uptake of radiolabelled antibodies[121] and could therefore improve the response to RIT. Increased uptake might be the result of increased blood flow, while improved response could be due to reduction in damage repair, and the toxic effect of heating on therapy-resistant hypoxic cells. The mechanisms are still under investigation, and the optimal hyperthermic schedule is yet to be described. For example, differences in biodistribution have been reported between two thermally equivalent regimens[122].

Combination of RIT with other therapeutic agents can lead to additive, or even synergistic, results. Examples of this include the use of vascular disrupting agents (VDAs), antiangiogenic molecules, and the hypoxia-selective cytotoxin tirapazamine. VDAs disrupt the structure of established tumour blood vessels. Combretastatin A4P (CA4P) is a tubulin-binding agent, and exerts at least part of its effect through disrupting the morphology of endothelial cells, leading to a rapid shutdown of tumour blood supply[123,124]. This results in necrosis of the more hypoxic, radioresistant centre of the tumour, but leaves a viable rim of tumour cells that will continue to grow. RIT is more effective in this well-perfused outer region of the tumour. Antibody administered before the CA4P is trapped in the radiosensitive rim of the tumour by the action of CA4P, increasing the dose to the outer region of tumour, while the action of CA4P itself results in massive central tumour necrosis[125,126]. This combination of therapies has been shown to lead to a greater than additive effect, and is currently being investigated in clinical trials. A second VDA, 5,6-dimethylxanthenone-4-acetic acid (DMXAA), has similarly been shown to enhance RIT[127], while an antiangiogenic therapy (2-methoxyestradiol) increased survival time in a colorectal liver metastasis model[128].

It has been reported that following RIT the tumour can become hypoxic. A regimen was tested to combine RIT with a therapy specifically toxic towards hypoxic cells. Combination of RIT with tirapazamine, given when the tumour was most hypoxic, resulted in an improvement in therapy[129]. Successful application of this type of combination depends on the reaction of the tissue to targeted radiotherapy and the pattern of oxygenation of the tissue, which is not predictable and has been demonstrated to vary significantly.

Once the antibody has left the blood vessel it must interact with the antigen in order to be retained at the tumour site. Antigen expression level and distribution also affect RIC uptake. Increasing the expression of antigen, leading to a twofold increase in antibody uptake, has been demonstrated using interferon[130,131]. Heterogeneous expression of antigen throughout the tumour might be overcome by using a cocktail of antibodies that are raised against different antigens expressed throughout the tumour, resulting in a more homogeneous distribution of dose[130]. Antigen expression level and distribution also affect RIC uptake. Interferon-γ has been reported[132] to increase tumour CEA expression and made TAG-72 (tumour-associated glycoprotein 72) distribution more homogeneous throughout the tumour, leading to higher localization of radioisotope.

2.5.2 Improvements to antibody delivery

The rate of clearance of the antibody from the circulation affects the extent of uptake at the tumour site, and therefore the total dose that can be delivered to the tumour. Efforts in this area have focused on altering normal tissue retention and the clearance and tumour site localization kinetics of the radionuclide.

Fast clearance of antibody from the blood reduces the amount that can localize to the tumour site. Where deiodination is limiting uptake, this can be reduced by use of a more stable, indirect labelling technique. Smaller antibody fragments, such as scFvs, are cleared rapidly from the blood via the kidneys, with catabolism further increasing normal tissue retention and therefore dose[133]. Administration of basic amino acids, such as lysine, has been reported to reduce accumulation of antibody in the kidney[134], enabling increased administration[133]. For large antibodies, where slow clearance rates result in low tumour to normal ratios, a secondary antibody reactive with the first could be given to increase the rate of clearance of the RIC from the blood[135,136]. In this situation, a greater initial dose of RIC can be delivered, and the clearing antibody given once sufficient radioisotope has localized to the tumour site. This results in less dose to the blood pool, reducing toxicity, and potentially give a higher initial dose rate to the tumour. Disadvantages of this technique include higher uptakes in the liver and spleen due to clearance of the resultant complexes through these organs, and that the RIC is not cleared from the extravascular space, just from the blood.

A more sophisticated approach to overcome systemic toxicity caused by the RIC is pretargeted RIT, or PRIT. First suggested in 1986[137,138] the basis of PRIT is to separate the administration of the antibody and the radioisotope. While a number of formats have been devised, varying in number of steps and exact protocol, the following description serves as an illustration. The antibody raised against tumour-specific antigen is labelled with a small molecule before being injected. Antibodies used in PRIT are chosen for their slow clearance from the blood, increasing tumour uptake. After a suitable period a clearing agent is used to remove any remainder from the blood and the radioisotope of choice, attached to a small molecule, which will react with that associated with the localized antibody, is administered. The nature of the smaller radioisotope vehicle means that it is quickly cleared from normal tissues, minimizing toxicity, while delivering therapy to the tumour. Avidin/biotin-based systems have dominated this area, and some clinical applications of RIT use this technology. For PRIT, doses and timings are critical. Problems with the avidin–biotin type procedures include the endogenous biotin (in the liver), the immunogenicity of streptavidin, antigen shedding and antibody internalization. Antibody engineering has been applied to produce a bispecific antibody which reacts with both the tumour and part of a hapten for the more advanced affinity enhancement system (for a review see reference 139).

2.5.3 Radiation

The measures described above increase delivery of the maximal amount of radioisotope to the tumour. The response of the tumour to radiotherapy is governed by the radiosensitivity of the cells, which can be modified by local environmental conditions such as oxygenation, as previously described. Hypoxia-selective toxins given in combination with RIT have conferred an advantage[129,140], suggesting that the hypoxic compartment contributes to therapeutic resistance. Although differences between the effect of the low-dose rate achieved in normoxic and hypoxic regions of tumours by RIT might be small, these studies suggest that they are significant.

Having discussed the basic components of RIT, how they interact and how the efficacy of RIT might be improved, we will now provide a representative selection of examples of how lessons learned at the preclinical level are being translated into clinical practice in early stage trials.

2.6 Clinical employment of radioimmunotherapy

Haematological malignancies are typically good targets for RIT, presenting a radiosensitive disseminated target with reduced barriers to access. Encouraging results have been obtained, especially with the CD20-targeting antibodies (for review see reference 141). Results for solid tumour types are less positive, with encouraging indications from preclinical models often difficult to replicate in the clinic. For the purposes of this introduction to RIT we will concentrate on its clinical application to solid tumours, specifically colorectal and brain tumours. These provide examples of the approaches that have been employed and how challenges to RIT are being overcome to further establish its place in the cancer therapy armoury.

2.6.1 Colorectal cancer

The majority of clinical trials targeting colorectal cancer have used ^{131}I and ^{90}Y, with a report of ^{177}Lu use[142], while antigens targeted include CEA (in the majority of cases), TAG-72, A33, Ep-CAM, and CSA-p. Bulky primary tumours rarely respond to RIT, so its application in the clinic has often been as a follow-up to surgical resection. The extensive blood supply linking the gut and liver leads to metastatic spread of the tumour to this organ. Metastatic deposits are often more difficult to address and can lead to therapy failure. This leads to the interesting conundrum that the results of trials using RIT against bulky large volume disease are often poor, but successful therapy in cases of small volume and occult disease are hard to quantify due to the limitations of detection in medical imaging. Site of injection might increase tumour localization of radionuclide while potentially decreasing toxicity. The following studies give examples of routes of administration, activities given, toxicity encountered, and positive results. In considering these studies, however, it must be remembered that colorectal cancer patients receiving RIT have been heavily pretreated with conventional therapeutics before entering the trials.

While whole antibodies have emerged as a mainstay of clinical RIT, the use of F(ab′)$_2$ fragments has also been reported[24,30]. In the former trial these were radiolabelled (^{131}I) and localization and therapy compared with the parent whole antibody (A5B7 IgG1 mAb). The F(ab′)$_2$ fragments localized more rapidly (8.2% injected activity (IA)/kg at 4.25 hours compared with 4.4% IA/kg for the whole mAb, $P < 0.05$), resulting in higher dose rates delivered by the smaller fragments, and responses were seen in both patient groups.

Higher dose to tumour is achieved in smaller lesions[14]. Encouraging results were obtained in a study deliberately focusing on small volume disease[143] treating 30 patients with lesions of ≤ 3.0 cm with 60 mCi/m^2 given as one dose of ^{131}I-LMN-14 IgG. An objective response rate of 16% and overall response of 58% (three partial responses and eight minor responses) was reported. In an adjuvant combination group (liver resection of metastases) seven of nine patients were free from disease for up to 36 months, whereas in an historical control group the relapse rate was 67%.

Clinical trials are usually at the phase I/II dose escalation stage and therefore have low doses, but sometimes higher doses with more therapeutic intent are used and require haematological support. High-dose RIT with autologous stem cell support has been reported[144]. A dose escalation from 50 to 300 mCi/m^2 using ^{131}I resulted in good tumour localization (%ID/g from 0.2–2.1), and absorbed dose from 630 to 3300 cGy. However, poorer localization and toxicity were reported when ^{90}Y was used. Heavily pretreated patients given escalating doses of ^{131}I-labelled anti-A33 antibody produced no objective results, the Maximum tolerated dose (MTD) being limited to 75 mCi/m^2.

A pretargeted study[145] employed the NR-LU-10 pancarcinoma antibody. The system used a streptavidin conjugate of the antibody with ^{90}Y-DOTA-biotin (given as 1×110 mCi/m^2), and achieved a modest overall response rate, with four patients (of 25) having freedom from progressive disease for 10–20 weeks.

The application of combined EBRT and RIT has been subject to a feasibility study[146]: ^{131}I-labelled anti-CEA mAb F(ab')$_2$ fragments (mean dose of 6.9 GBq) and 20 Gy RT to the liver were given in quick succession, this being the optimal protocol indicated by preclinical studies. While myelotoxicity and liver toxicity were encountered, a minor response was reported in one patient and stable disease in three others (of six).

Dose fractionation can lead to lower toxicity for the same administered total dose[147]. The chimeric IgG4 antibody B72.3 was given in two or three doses to a total of 28 or 36 mCi/m^2. Lower bone marrow toxicity was reported than for the same dose given as a single administration ($P = 0.04$). For further discussion of this approach see reference 148.

As an alternative route of administration to i.v. intrahepatic arterial infusion has been tested against colorectal metastases[24], but localization was similar to that seen following introduction into a peripheral vein. However, it is possible that an advantage could be gained if a high-affinity antibody with rapid antigen binding were employed. Encouraging results were obtained when this technique was used against hepatocellular carcinoma[149]. Long-term survival was improved compared with a resection only group (28.1% compared with 9.1%, $P < 0.05$). Locoregional administration (i.p.)[150] has demonstrated higher uptake in metastatic carcinoma in the peritoneum, whereas i.v. administration targeted lymph nodes and local recurrences more effectively.

As well as combining RIT with irradiative therapy, the option to add chemotherapy to the regimen has been explored[151]. Up to three cycles of a ^{90}Y-labelled anti-CEA antibody was given (16.6 mCi/m^2) to patients with chemotherapy-refractory metastatic cancer. This was combined with 5-fluorouracil (700–1000 mg/m^2/day for 5 days), the combination being given for up to three cycles. This therapy did not increase 5-fluorouracil associated toxicity, and achieved stable disease in 11 of 21 patients for 3–8 months. Repeat administration of the antibody was possible in most cases, whereas it had been precluded by immunogenic reactions in previous studies, and the authors suggest that the addition of 5-fluorouracil reduced the HACA response.

2.6.2 Brain cancer

As with the colorectal clinical trials, most brain-targeted RIT focuses on the use of whole antibodies, tenascin being the main antigen targeted. While some studies have used systemic (intravenous or intra-arterial) administration of antibody, more recent reports have tended to move towards local administration. This is for a number of reasons: antitenascin antibodies can have high uptake in the liver and spleen when injected i.v., increasing normal tissue toxicity; access to the brain can be reduced by the blood–brain barrier, which might still be at least partially intact; it is desirable to limit dose delivered to normal brain as much as possible; disease of the brain and CNS lends itself to locoregoinal administration, through intrathecal (i.e. into the cerebrospinal fluid bathing the spinal cord and brain) or intra cavity (following surgery) introduction, maximizing the effect on residual cells. Local recurrence is a problem with tumours of the brain. There is evidence that cellular invasion does not generally extend far from the rim of the disease site (e.g. < 2 cm)[142,153]. Limited extension of disease into surrounding normal brain is an important factor in successful application of RIT in this context[154]. These reports of clinical trials illustrate different techniques that have been investigated and major findings.

Following imaging and confirmation of antibody localization selected patients with brain glioma were treated with 40–140 mCi of ^{131}I-labelled antibody given either intravenously or via the carotid artery[155]. There was no major toxicity reported, and six patients (of 10) showed clinical improvement lasting from 6 months to 3 years. The route of administration made no difference to tumour localization, as has been reported elsewhere[156].

A single dose of ^{131}I-labelled 81C6 antibody (antitenascin) was given intrathecally to patients with leptomeningeal neoplasms or brain tumour resection cavities[157]. Haematological toxicity was dose limiting. The MTD in adults was found to be 80 mCi. Of 31 patients there was one partial response, 13 stabilizations of disease and favourable long-term survival rates.

A study involving both recurrent and newly diagnosed cases of malignant gliomas again gave ^{131}I-labelled antitenascin antibody using a surgically implanted in-dwelling catheter[158]. Little systemic or cerebral toxicity was reported, and administered doses escalated from 185 to 2405 MBq for up to six cycles. High uptake in neoplastic tissue and long retention resulted in doses delivered to tumour of >30 000 cGy. The median survival was 20 months, 18 for recurrent cases and 23 in newly diagnosed. A later report gives a response rate of 51.6%, including nine partial responses, three complete response, and 20 (of 62) no evidence of disease (NED)[154].

In a study 24 patients with recurrent glioma, consisting of eight with anaplastic astrocytoma and 16 with glioblastoma, were treated with ^{90}Y PRIT[159]. Following secondary surgery and surgical introduction of a catheter the patients were admistered 2 mg antitenascin mAb directly into the cavity, followed after 24 hours with avidin, then finally 18 hours later ^{90}Y-labelled biotin. Stable disease was achieved in 50% of patients (seven glioblastoma and five anaplastic astrocytoma), and an objective response was observed in 25% of patients at an administered dose of 0.7–0.9 GBq. The MTD was limited by neurological toxicity to 30 mCi, with no acute toxicity up to 20 mCi. In a follow-up study[160] 73 patients with glioblastoma were treated with either locoregional RIT alone ($n = 38$) or in combination with temozolomide ($n = 35$). RIT was given using a three-step form of ^{90}Y pretargeting, administered using a catheter introduced during the secondary surgery following recurrence. The amount of activity given varied according to cavity volume rather than amount of tumour remaining, ranging from 370 to 925 MBq, in two to seven cycles. RIT alone resulted in a median overall survival of 17.5 months and a progression-free survival of 5 months. In combination with temozolomide, chosen for its complementary activity to irradiative therapy, median overall survival was extended to 25 months and progression-free survival to 10 months, with no additional neurotoxicity or major haemotoxicity. While this was not a randomized study the results do suggest an advantage in combining RIT with chemotherapy.

The cases reported above demonstrate how RIT has been employed in a manner that capitalizes on its strengths. The progression towards RIT given to treat minimal disseminated disease in colorectal cancer patients is clear, and results are encouraging. Similarly, the treatment of brain tumours following surgery, at a time when few tumour cells remain, has also produced encouraging results, even at this early dose escalation stage, with limited toxicity. Owing to the size of trial populations to date, their often advanced stage of disease, and the effects of previous therapies on patients, it can be difficult to directly compare studies and interpret data meaningfully. However, these studies show that RIT can indeed work, especially when used in concert with other therapeutic approaches.

2.7 Conclusions

In this introduction to RIT we have discussed this developing technique in three sections. Initially its three basic components, tumour, antibody, and radioisotope, were considered, and their relevant properties and inter-relationships described. Building on these concepts, we then demonstrated how some of the methods to improve RIT efficacy have been investigated. Finally, examples of the clinical application of RIT and results obtained were reported. The application of RIT as an adjuvant, against residual disease or small disseminated metastases, with appropriate administration and with steps taken to reduce exposure of normal tissues, appears to maximize its antitumour effects.

These case studies have provided very promising results that offer much hope for the future. RIT clearly has the potential to contribute significantly in the on-going struggle to successfully treat common solid tumours.

2.7.1 **Summary**

RIT is a technique in which a therapeutic isotope is delivered specifically to tumour cells. The nuclide is attached to an antibody raised against molecules expressed predominantly on the surface of the target tumour cells. The antibody and nuclide (or RIC) clear from normal tissues but localize to, and are retained in, the tumour by antigen binding.

The three principal factors in RIT are the tumour, the antibody, and the radionuclide.

1. *Tumour*
   - must express antigen at sufficient levels for localization and higher than normal tissues for specific uptake
   - tumour size will influence uptake—smaller tumours have higher uptake
   - tumour site could guide route of administration for maximal effect.

2. *Antibody*
   - affinity (a measure of the strength of antigen binding) is important for tumour localization and retention
   - size will affect clearance and tumour penetration
   - immunogenicity will influence clearance and retreatment

3. *Radioisotope*
   - chemistry should be amenable to antibody conjugation
   - emissions will define the biological effect
   - physical half-life should allow for time taken to localize to, and retention at, tumour site
   - maximum radiation dose administered is usually limited by bone marrow toxicity

Acknowledgements

The authors wish to thank Dr Alexandra Huhalov for useful discussions and preparation. Work in the Department of Oncology, Royal Free & UCL Medical School is supported by Cancer Research UK, European Union FP 6 Project Number LSHC-CT-2003-503233 STROMA and NTRAC.

References

1. Jain RK (1999). Transport of molecules, particles, and cells in solid tumors. *Annual Review of Biomedical Engineering* **1**: 241–63.
2. Vogel C-A, Galmiche MC, Westermann P, Sun L-Q, Pelegrin A, Folli S, Bischoff Delaloye A, Slosman DO, Mach J-P, Buchegger F (1996). Carcinoembryonic antigen expression, antibody localisation and immunophotodetection of human colon cancer

liver metastases in nude mice: A model for radioimmunotherapy. *International Journal of Cancer* **67**: 294–302.

3. Dearling JLJ, Qureshi U, Whiting S, Boxer GM, Begent RHJ, Pedley RB (2005). Analysis of antibody distribution reveals higher uptake in peripheral intrahepatic deposits than central deposits. *European Journal of Nuclear Medicine and Molecular Imaging* **32**: S83.

4. Gold P, Freedman SO (1965). Specific carcinoembryonic antigens of the human digestive system. *Journal of Experimental Medicine* **122**: 467–481.

5. Benchimol S, Fuks A, Jothy S, Beauchemin N, Shirota K, Stanners CP (1989). Carcinoembryonic antigen, a human tumor marker, functions as an intercellular adhesion molecule. *Cell* **57**: 327–34.

6. Tibbetts LM, Doremus CM, Tzanakis GN, Vezeridis MP (1993). Liver metastases with 10 human colon carcinoma cell lines in nude mice and association with carcinoembryonic antigen production. *Cancer* **71**: 315–21.

7. Toth CA, Rapoza A, Zamcheck N, Steele G, Thomas P (1989). Receptor-mediated endocytosis of carcinoembryonic antigen by rat alveolar macrophages *in vitro*. *Journal of Leukocyte Biology* **45**: 370–6.

8. Sung C, Shockley TR, Morrison PF, Dvorak HF, Yarmush ML, Dedrick RL (1992). Predicted and observed effects of antibody affinity and antigen density on monoclonal antibody uptake in solid tumors. *Cancer Research* **52**: 377–84.

9. Goldenberg A, Masui H, Divgi C, Kamrath H, Pentlow K, Mendelsohn J (1989). Imaging of human tumor xenografts with an indium-111-labelled anti-epidermal growth factor receptor monoclonal antibody. *Journal of the National Cancer Institute* **81**: 1616–25.

10. Humm JL, Cobb LM (1990). Nonuniformity of tumor dose in radioimmunotherapy. *Journal of Nuclear Medicine* **31**: 75–83.

11. Humm JL, Chin LM, Cobb LM, Begent RHJ (1990). Microdosimetry in radioimmunotherapy. *Radiation Protection Dosimetry* **31**: 433–6.

12. Quayle JB (1982). Ability of CEA blood levels to reflect tumour burden: a study in a human xenograft model. *British Journal of Cancer* **46**: 220–7.

13. Pedley RB, Boden JA, Boden RW, Green A, Boxer GM, Bagshawe KD (1989). The effect of serum CEA on the distribution and clearance of anti-CEA antibody in a pancreatic tumour xenograft model. *British Journal of Cancer* **60**: 549–54.

14. Behr TM, Sharkey RM, Juweid MI, Dunn RM, Ying Z, Zhang C-H, Siegel JA, Gold DV, Goldenberg DM (1996). Factors influencing the pharmacokinetics, dosimetry, and diagnostic accuracy of radioimmunodetection and radioimmunotherapy of carcinoembrynic antigen-expressing tumors. *Cancer Research* **56**: 1805–16.

15. Kohler G, Milstein C (1975). Continuous cultures of fused cells secreting antibody of predefined specificity. *Nature* **256**: 495–7.

16. Clark M, Cobbold S, Hale G, *et al.* (1983). Advantages of rat monoclonal antibodies. *Immunology Today* **4**: 100–1.

17. McCafferty J, Griffiths AD, Winter G, Chiswell DJ (1990). Phage antibodies: filamentous phage displaying antibody variable domains. *Nature* **348**: 552–4.

18. Maynard J, Georgiou G (2000). Antibody engineering. *Annual Review of Biomedical Engineering* **2**: 339–76.

19. Yazaki PJ, Shively L, Clark C, Cheung CW, Le W, Szpikowska B, Shively JE, Raubitschek AA, Wu AM (2001). Mammalian expression and hollow fiber bioreactor

production of recombinant anti-CEA diabody and minibody for clinical applications. *Journal of Immunological Methods* **253:** 195–208.

20. de Graaf M, van der Meulen-Muileman IH, Pinedo HM, Haisma HJ (2002). Expression of scFvs and scFv fusion proteins in eukaryotic cells. *Methods Mol Biol* **178:** 379–87.

21. Houdebine LM (2002). Antibody manufacture in transgenic animals and comparisons with other systems. *Curret Opinion in Biotechnology* **13:** 625–9.

22. Stoger E, Sack M, Fischer R, Christou P (2002). Plantibodies: applications, advantages and bottlenecks. *Curret Opinion in Biotechnology* **13:** 161–6.

23. Buchegger F, Pelegrin A, Delaloye B, Bischof-Delaloye A, Mach JP (1990). Iodine-131-labelled MAb F(ab')2 fragments are more efficient and less toxic than intact anti-CEA antibodies in radioimmunotherapy of large human colon carcinoma grafted in nude mice. *Journal of Nuclear Medicine* **31:** 1035–44.

24. Buchegger F, Gillet M, Doenz F, *et al.* (1996). Biodistribution of anti-CEA F(ab')2 fragments after intra-arterial and intravenous injection in patients with liver metastases due to colorectal carcinoma. *Nuclear Medicine Communications* **17:** 500–3.

25. Behr TM, Blumenthal RD, Memtsoudis S, *et al.* (2000). Cure of metastatic human colonic cancer in mice with radiolabeled monoclonal antibody fragments. *Clinical Cancer Research* **6:** 4900–7.

26. Casey JL, Pedley RB, King DJ, Green AJ, Yarranton GT, Begent RHJ (1999). Dosimetric evaluation and radioimmunotherapy of anti-tumour multivalent Fab' fragments. *British Journal of Cancer* **81:** 972–80.

27. Casey JL, Napier MP, King DJ, Pedley RB, Chaplin LC, Weir N, Skelton L, Green AJ, Hope-Stone LD, Yarranton GT, Begent RH (2002). Tumour targeting of humanised cross-linked divalent-Fab' antibody fragments: a clinical phase I/II study. *British Journal of Cancer* **86:** 1401–10.

28. Donda A, Cesson V, Mach JP, Corradin G, Primus FJ, Robert B (2003). *In vivo* targeting of an anti-tumour antibody coupled to antigenic MHC class I complexes induces specific growth inhibition and regression of established syngeneic tumor grafts. *Cancer Immunity* **3:** 11.

29. Pastorino F, Brignole C, Marimpietri D, Sapra P, Moase EH, Allen TM, Ponzoni M (2003). Doxorubicin-loaded Fab' fragments of anti-disialoganglioside immunoliposomes selectively inhibit the growth and dissemination of human neuroblasotma in nude mice. *Cancer Research* **63:** 86–92.

30. Lane DM, Eagle,KF, Begent, RH, *et al.* (1994). Radioimmunotherapy of metastatic colorectal tumours with iodine-131-labelled antibody to carcinoembryonic antigen: phase I/II study with comparative biodistribution of intact and F(ab')2 antibodies. *British Journal of Cancer* **70:** 521–5.

31. Huston JS, Levinson D, Mudgett-Hunter M, *et al.* (1988). Protein engineering of antibody binding sites: recovery of specific activity in an anti-digoxin single-chain Fv analogue produced in *Escherichia coli. Proceedings of the National Academy of Sciences USA* **85:** 5879–83.

32. Bird RE, Hardman KD, Jacobson JW, *et al.* (1988). Single-chain antigen-binding proteins. *Science* **242:** 423–6.

33. Colcher D, Bird R, Roselli M, *et al.* (1990). In vivo tumor targeting of a recombinant single-chain antigen-binding protein. *Journal of the National Cancer Institute* **82:** 1191–7.

34. Milenic DE, Yokota T, Filpula DR, *et al.* (1991). Construction, binding properties, metabolism, and tumor targeting of a single-chain Fv derived from the pancarcinoma monoclonal antibody CC49. *Cancer Research* **51:** 6363–71.

35. Yokota T, Milenic DE, Whitlow M, Schlom J (1992). Rapid tumor penetration of a single-chain Fv and comparison with other immunoglobulin forms. *Cancer Research* **52:** 3402–8.

36. Yokota T, Milenic DE, Whitlow M, Wood JF, Hubert SL, Schlom J (1993). Microautoradiographic analysis of the normal organ distribution of radioiodinated single-chain Fv and other immunoglobulin forms. *Cancer Research* **53:** 3776–83.

37. Adams GP, McCartney JE, Tai MS, *et al.* (1993). Highly specific in vivo tumor targeting by monovalent and divalent forms of 741F8 anti-c-erbB-2 single-chain Fv. *Cancer Research* **53:** 4026–34.

38. Begent RH, Verhaar MJ, Chester KA, *et al.* (1996). Clinical evidence of efficient tumor targeting based on single-chain Fv antibody selected from a combinatorial library. *Nature Medicine* **2:** 979–84.

39. Larson SM, El Shirbiny AM, Divgi CR, *et al.* (1997). Single chain antigen binding protein (sFv CC49): first human studies in colorectal carcinoma metastatic to liver. *Cancer* **80:** 2458–68.

40. Pavlinkova G, Beresford G, Booth BJ, Batra SK, Colcher D (1999). Charge-modified single chain antibody constructs of monoclonal antibody CC49: generation, characterisation, pharmacokinetics, and bioditribution analysis. *Nuclear Medicine and Biology* **26:** 27–34.

41. Michael NP, Chester KA, Melton RG, *et al.* (1996). In vitro and in vivo characterisation of a recombinant carboxypeptidase G2::anti-CEA scFv fusion protein. *Immunotechnology* **2:** 47–57.

42. Bhatia J, Sharma SK, Chester KA, *et al.* (2000). Catalytic activity of an in vivo tumor targeted anti-CEA scFv::carboxypeptidase G2 fusion protein. *International Journal of Cancer* **85:** 571–7.

43. Cooke SP, Pedley RB, Boden R, Begent RH, Chester KA (2002). In vivo tumor delivery of a recombinant single chain Fv::tumor necrosis factor-alpha fusion protein. *Bioconjugate Chemistry* **13:** 7–15.

44. Huhalov A, Chester KA (2004). Engineered single chain antibody fragments for radioimmunotherapy. *Quarterly Journal of Nuclear Medicine and Molecular Imaging* **48:** 279–88.

45. Schlom J, Eggensperger D, Colcher D, *et al.* (1992). Therapeutic advantage of high-affinity anticarcinoma radioimmunoconjugates. *Cancer Research* **52:** 1067–72.

46. Colcher D, Minelli MF, Roselli M, Muraro R, Simpson-Milenic D, Schlom J (1988). Radioimmunolocalisation of human carcinoma xenografts with B72.3 second generation monoclonal antibodies. *Cancer Research* **48:** 4597–603.

47. Kuan C-T, Wikstrand CJ, Archer G, *et al.* (2000). Increased binding affinity enhances targeting of glioma xenografts by EGFRVIII-specific scFv. *International Journal of Cancer* **88:** 962–9.

48. Muraro R, Kuroki M, Wunderlich D *et al.* (1988). Generation and characterisation of B72.3 second generation monoclonal antibodies reactive with the tumor-associated glycoprotein 72 antigen. *Cancer Research* **48:** 4588–96.

49. Adams GP, Schier R, Marshall K, *et al.* (1998). Increased affinity leads to improved selective tumor delivery of single-chain Fv antibodies. *Cancer Research* **58:** 485–90.

50. Behr TM, Sharkey RM, Juweid ME, *et al.* (1997). Variables influencing tumor dosimetry in radioimmunotherapy of CEA-expressing cancers with anti-CEA and anti-mucin monoclonal antibodies. *Journal of Nuclear Medicine* **38:** 409–18.

51. van Osdol W, Fujimori K, Weinstein JN (1991). An analysis of monoclonal antibody distribution in microscopic tumor nodules: consequences of a 'binding site barrier'. *Cancer Research* **51:** 4776–84.

52. Saga T, Neumann RD, Heya T, *et al.* (1995). Targeting cancer micrometastases with monoclonal antibodies: A binding-site barrier. *Proceedings of the National Academy of Sciences USA* **92:** 8999–9003.

53. Karush F (1970). Affinity and the immune response. *Annals of the New York Academy of Sciences* **169:** 56–64.

54. Adams GP, McCartney JE, Wolf EJ, *et al.* (1995). Enhanced tumor specificity of 741F8-1 (sFv′)2, an anti-c-erbB-2 single-chain Fv dimer, mediated by stable radioiodine conjugation. *Journal of Nuclear Medicine* **36:** 2276–81.

55. Goel A, Colcher D, Baranowska-Kortylewicz J, *et al.* (2001). 99mTc-labeled divalent and tetravalent CC49 single-chain Fv's: novel imaging agents for rapid *in vivo* localisation of human colon carcinoma. *Journal of Nuclear Medicine* **42:** 1519–27.

56. Todorovska A, Roovers RC, Dolezal O, Kortt AA, Hoogenboom HR, Hudson PJ (2001). Design and application of diabodies, triabodies and tetrabodies for cancer imaging. *Journal of Immunological Methods* **248:** 47–66.

57. Mirick GR, Bradt BM, Denardo SJ, Denardo GL (2004). A review of human anti-globulin antibody (HAGA, HAMA, HACA, HAHA) responses to monoclonal antibodies. Not four letter words. *Quarterly Journal of Nuclear Medicine and Molecular Imaging* **48:** 251–7.

58. Mendez MJ, Green LL, Corvalan JR, *et al.* (1997). Functional transplant of megabase human immunoglobulin loci recapitulates human antibody response in mice. *Nature Genetics* **15:** 146–56.

59. Nagy ZA, Hubner B, Lohning C *et al.* (2002). Fully human, HLA-DR-specific monoclonal antibodies efficiently induce programmed death of malignant lymphoid cells. *Nature Medicine* **8:** 801–7.

60. O'Connell D, Becerril B, Roy-Burman A, *et al.* (2002). Phage versus phagemid libraries for generation of human monoclonal antibodies. *Journal of Molecular Biology* **321:** 49–56.

61. Knappik A, Ge L, Honegger A, *et al.* (2000). Fully synthetic human combinatorial antibody libraries (HuCAL) based on modular consensus frameworks and CDRs randomised with trinucleotides. *Journal of Molecular Biology* **296:** 57–86.

62. Pederson JT, Henry AH, Searle SJ, *et al.* (1994). Comparison of surface accessible residues in human and murine immunoglobulin Fv domains. Implication for humanization of murine antibodies. *Journal of Molecular Biology* **235:** 959–73.

63. Roguska MA, Pederson JT, Keddy CA, *et al.* (1994). Humanization of murine monoclonal antibodies through variable domain resurfacing. *Proceedings of the National Academy of Sciences USA* **91:** 969–73.

64. Hofer KG (1996). Biophysical aspects of Auger processes. *Acta Oncologica* **35:** 789–96.

65. Imam SK (2001). Advancements in cancer therapy with alpha-emitters: A review. *International Journal of Radiation Oncology, Biology, Physics* **51:** 271–8.

66. Zalutsky MR, Vaidyanathan G (2000). Astatine-211-labelled radiotherapeutics: An emerging approach to targeted alpha-particle radiotherapy. *Current Pharmaceutical Design* **6**: 1433–55.

67. McDevitt MR, Sgouros G, Finn RD, *et al.* (1998). Radioimmunotherapy with alpha-emitting nuclides. *European Journal of Nuclear Medicine* **25**: 1341–51.

68. Akabani G, McLendon RE, Bigner DD, Zalutsky MR (2002). Vascular targeted endoradiotherapy of tumors using alpha-particle-emitting compounds: Theoretical analysis. *International Journal of Radiation Oncology, Biology, Physics* **54**: 1259–75.

69. Akabani G, Kennel SJ, Zalutsky MR (2003). Microdosimetric analysis of α-particle-emitting targeted radiotherapeutics using histological images. *Journal of Nuclear Medicine* **44**: 792–805.

70. Simpkin DJ, Mackie TR (1990). EGS4 Monte Carlo determination of the beta dose kernel in water. *Medical Physics* **17**(2): 179–86.

71. Flynn AA, Green AJ, Pedley RB, *et al.* (2002). A model-based approach for the optimization of radioimmunotherapy through antibody design and radionuclide selection. *Cancer* **94**: 1249–57.

72. O'Donoghue JA, Bardies M, Wheldon TE (1995). Relationships between tumor size and curability for uniformly targted therapy with beta-emitting radionuclides *Journal of Nuclear Medicine* **36**: 1902–9.

73. Howell RW, Goddu SM, Rao DV (1998). Proliferation and the advantage of longer- lived radionuclides in radioimmunotherapy. *Medical Physics* **25**; 37–42.

74. Greenwood FC, Hunter WM (1963). The preparation of ^{131}I-labelled human growth hormone of high specific radioactivity. *Biochemistry Journal* **89**: 116–23.

75. Verel I, Visser GWM, Vosjan MJWD, Finn R, Boellaard R, van Dongen GAMS (2004). High-quality ^{124}I-labelled monoclonal antibodies for use as PET scouting agents prior to ^{131}I-radioimmunotherapy. *European Journal of Nuclear Medicine and Molecular Imaging* **31**: 1645–52.

76. Bolton AE, Hunter WM (1973). The labelling of proteins to a I-125 containing acylating agent. *Biochemical Journal* **133**: 529–39.

77. Zalutsky MR, Noska MA, Colapinto EV, Garg PK, Bigner DD (1989). Enhanced tumor localisation and in vivo stability of a monoclonal antibody radioiodinated using N-succinimidyl 3-(tri-n-butylstannyl)benzoate. *Cancer Research* **49**: 5543–9.

78. Shankar S, Vaidyanathan G, Affleck D, Welsh PC, Zalutsky MR (2003). *N*-Succinimidyl 3-[^{131}I]Iodo-4-phosphonomethylbenzoate ([^{131}I]SIPMB), a negatively charged substituent-bearing acylation agent for the radioiodination of peptides and mAbs. *Bioconjugate Chemistry* **14**: 331–41.

79. Wilbur DS, Hadley SW, Hylarides MD, Abrams PG, Beaumier PA, Morgan AC, Reno JM, Fritzberg AR (1989). Development of a stable radioiodinating reagent to label monoclonal antibodies for radiotherapy of cancer. *Journal of Nuclear Medicine* **30**: 216–26.

80. Stein R, Goldenberg DM, Thorpe SR, Basu A, Mattes MJ (1995). Effects of radiolabelling monoclonal antibodies with a residualising iodine radiolabel on the accretion of radioisotope in tumours. *Cancer Research* **55**: 3132–9.

81. Hagan PL, Halpern SE, Dillman RO, *et al.* (1986). Tumor size: effect on monoclonal antibody uptake in tumor models. *Journal of Nuclear Medicine* **27**: 422–7.

82. Pedley RB, Boden J, Keep PA, Harwood PJ, Green AJ, Begent RHJ (1987). Relationship between tumour size and uptake of radiolabelled anti-CEA in a colon tumour xenograft. *European Journal of Nuclear Medicine* **13**: 197–202.

83. Mayer A, Tsiompanou E, Flynn AA, *et al.* (2003). Higher dose and dose-rate in smaller tumors result in improved control. *Cancer Investigation* **21**: 382–8.

84. Verel I, Visser GWM, Boellaard R *et al.* (2003). Quantitative ^{89}Zr immuno-PET for *in vivo* scouting of ^{90}Y-labeled monoclonal antibodies in xenograft-bearing nude mice. *Journal of Nuclear Medicine* **44**: 1663–70.

85. Williams LE, Lui A, Wu AM, Odom-Maryon T, Chai A, Raubitschek AA, Wong JYC (1995). Figures of merit (FOMs) for imaging and therapy using monoclonal antibodies *Medical Physics* **22**(12): 2025–7.

86. Dale RG (1996). Dose-rate effects in targeted radiotherapy. *Physics in Medicine Biology* **41**: 1871–84.

87. Denekamp J, Waites T, Fowler JF (1997). Predicting realistic RBE values for clinically relevant radiotherapy schedules. *International Journal of Radiation Biology* **71**: 681–94.

88. Langmuir VK, Fowler JF, Knox SJ, Wessels BW, Sutherland RM, Wong JYC (1993). Radiobiology of radiolabelled antibody therapy as applied to tumor dosimetry. *Medical Physics* **20**(2): 601–10.

89. Juweid ME (2002). Radioimmunotherapy of B-cell non-Hodgkin's lymphoma: from clinical trials to clinical practice. *Journal of Nuclear Medicine* **43**: 1507–29.

90. Hall EJ (2000). *Radiobiology for the radiobiologist* (5th edn). Philadelphia, PA: Lippincott Williams & Wilkins.

91. Knox SJ, Goris ML, Wessels BW (1992). Overview of animal studies comparing radioimmunotherapy with dose equivalent external beam irradiation. *Radiotherapy and Oncology* **23**: 111–17.

92. Wessels BW, Vessela RL, Palme DF, Berkopec JM, Smith GK, Bradley EW (1989). Radiobiological comparison of external beam irradiation and radioimmunotherapy in renal cell carcinoma xenografts. *International Journal of Radiation Oncology, Biology, Physics* **17**: 1257–63.

93. Buchsbaum DJ, Ten Haken RK, Heidorn DB, Lawrence TS, Glatfelter AA, Terry VH, Guilbault DM, Steplewski Z, Lichter AS (1990). A comparison of 131I-labeled monoclonal antibody 17-1A treatment to external beam irradiation on the growth of LS174T human colon carcinoma xenografts. *International Journal of Radiation Oncology, Biology, Physics* **18**: 1033–41.

94. Williams JA, Edwards JA, Dillehay LE. (1992). Quantitative comparison of radiolabeled antibody therapy and external beam radiotherapy in the treatment of human glioma xenografts. *International Journal of Radiation Oncology, Biology, Physics* **24**: 111–17.

95. Buras RR, Wong JYC, Kuhn JA, Beatty BG, Williams LE, Wanek PM, Beatty JD (1993). Comparison of radioimmunotherapy in colon cancer xenografts. *International Journal of Radiation Oncology, Biology, Physics* **25**: 473–9.

96. Fowler JF (1990). Radiobiological aspects of low dose rates in radioimmunotherapy. *International Journal of Radiation Oncology, Biology, Physics* **18**: 1261–9.

97. Teicher BA (1994). Hypoxia and drug resistance. *Cancer and Metastasis Reviews* **13**: 139–68.

98. Trotter MJ, Chaplin DJ, Durand RE, Olive PL (1989). The use of fluorescent probes to identify regions of transient perfusion in murine tumors. *International Journal of Radiation Oncology, Biology, Physics* **16**: 931–4.

99. Palcic B, Brosing JW, Skarsgard LD (1982). Survival measurements at low doses: oxygen enhancement ratio. *British Journal of Cancer* **46**: 980–4.

100. Palcic B, Skarsgard LD (1984). Reduced oxygen enhancement ratio at low doses of ionizing radiation. *Radiation Research* **100**: 328–39.

101. Skarsgard LD, Harrison I (1991). Dose dependence of the oxygen enhancement ratio (OER) in radiation inactivation of Chinese hamster V79-171 cells. *Radiation Research* **127**: 243–7.

102. Hering ER, Sealy GRH, Dowman P, Blekkenhorst G (1987). OER and RBE for ^{125}I and ^{192}Ir at low dose rate on mammalian cells. *Radiotherapy and Oncology* **10**: 247–52.

103. Spiro IJ, Ling CC, Stickler, Gaskill (1985). Oxygen radiosensitisation at low dose rate. *British Journal of Radiology* **58**: 357–63.

104. Ling CC, Spiro IJ, Mitchell J, Stickler R (1985). The variation of OER with dose rate. *International Journal of Radiation Oncology, Biology, Physics* **11**: 1367–73.

105. O'Hara JA, Blumenthal RD, Grinberg OY, Demidenko E, Grinberg S, Wilmot CM, Taylor AM, Goldenberg DM, Swartz HM (2001). Response to radioimmunotherapy correlates with tumor pO_2 measured by EPR oximetry in human tumor xenografts. *Radiation Research* **155**: 466–73.

106. Morton JD, Porter E, Yabuki H, Nath R, Rockwell S (1990). Effects of a perfluorochemical emulsion on the response of BA1112 rat rhabdomyosarcomas to continuous low dose-rate irradiation. *Radiation Research* **124**: 178–82.

107. Sgouros G (1995). Radioimmunotherapy of micrometastases: Sidestepping the solid-tumor hurdle. *Journal of Nuclear Medicine* **36**: 1910–12.

108. Thames HD, Withers HR, Peters LJ (1984). Tissue repair capacity and repair kinetics deduced from multi-fractionated or continuous irradiation regimes with incomplete repair. *British Journal of Cancer* **49**: 263–9.

109. Muthaswamy MS, Roberson PL, Buchsbaum DJ (1998). A mouse bone marrow dosimetry model. *Journal of Nuclear Medicine* **39**: 1243–7.

110. Press OW, Eary JF, Appelbaum FR *et al.* (1993). Radiolabeled-antibody therapy of B-cell lymphoma with autologous bone marrow support. *New England Journal Medicine* **329**: 1219–24.

111. Morton BA, Beatty BG, Mison AP, Wanek PM, Beatty JD (1990). Role of bone marrow transplantation in 90Y antibody therapy of colon cancer in nude mice. *Cancer Research* **50**: 1008–10s.

112. Blumenthal RD, Alisauskas R, Lew W, Sharkey RM, Goldenberg DM (1998). Myelosuppressive changes from single or repeated doses of radioantibody therapy: effect of bone marrow transplantation, cytokines, and hematopoietic suppression. *Experimental Hematology* **26**: 859–68.

113. Blumenthal RD, Sharkey RM, Goldenberg DM (1992). Dose escalation of radioantibody in a mouse model with the use of recombinant human interleukin-1 and granulocyte-macrophage colony-stimulating factor intervention to reduce myelosuppression. *Journal of the National Cancer Institute* **84**: 399–407.

114. Vriesendorp HM, Shao Y, Blum JE, Quadri SM, Williams JR (1993). Fractionated intravenous administration of ^{90}Y-labeled B72.3 GYK-DTPA immunoconjugate in beagle dogs. *Nuclear Medicine and Biology* **20:** 571–8.

115. Pedley RB, Boden JA, Boden R, Dale R, Begent RH (1993). Comparative radioimmunotherapy using intact or F(ab')2 fragments of ^{131}I anti-CEA antibody in a colonic xenograft model. *British Journal of Cancer* **68:** 69–73.

116. Beaumier PL, Venkatesan P, Vanderheyden J-L, Burgua WD, Kunz LL, Fritzberg AR, Abrams PG, Morgan AC (1991). ^{186}Re Radioimmunotherapy of small cell lung carcinoma xenografts in nude mice. *Cancer Research* **51:** 676–81.

117. Goel A, Augustine S, Baranowska-Kortyewicz J, Colcher D, Booth BJM, Pavlinkova, Tempero M, Batra SK (2001). Single-dose versus fractionated radioimmunotherapy of human colon carcinoma xenografts using ^{131}I-labeled multivalent CC49 single-chain Fvs. *Clinical Cancer Research* **7:** 175–84.

118. Buchsbaum D, Khazaelli MB, Liu T, Bright S, Richardson K, Jones M, Meredith R (1995). Fractionated radioimmunotherapy of human colon carcinoma xenografts with ^{131}I-labeled monoclonal antibody CC49. *Cancer Research* **55:** 5881–7s.

119. Schlom J, Molinolo A, Simpson JF, Siler K, Roselli M, Hinkle G, Houchens DP, Colcher D (1990). Advantage of dose fractionation in monoclonal antibody-directed radioimmunotherapy. *Journal of the National Cancer Institute* **82:** 763–71.

120. Buchsbaum DJ, Khazaelli MB, Mayo MS, Roberson PL (1999). Comparison of multiple bolus and continuous injections of ^{131}I-labeled CC49 for therapy in a colon cancer xenograft model. *Clinical Cancer Research* **5:** 3153–9s.

121. Cope DA, Dewhirst MW, Friedman HS, Bigner DD, Zalutsky MR (1990). Enhanced delivery of a monoclonal antibody F(ab')2 fragment to subcutaneous human glioma xenografts using local hyperthermia. *Cancer Research* **50:** 1803–9.

122. Hauck ML, Zalutsky MR (2005). Enhanced tumour uptake of radiolabelled antibodies by hyperthermia. Part II: Application of the thermal equivalency equation. *International Journal of Hyperthermia* **21:** 13–27.

123. Thorpe PE (2004). Vascular targeting agents as cancer therapeutics. *Clinical Cancer Research* **10:** 415–27.

124. Tozer GM, Kanthou C, Baguley BC (2005). Disrupting tumour blood vessels. *Nature Reviews Cancer* **5:** 423–35.

125. Pedley RB, Hill SA, Boxer GM, *et al.* (2001). Eradication of colorectal xenografts by combined radioimmunotherapy and combretastatin A-4 3-O-phosphate. *Cancer Research* **61:** 4716–22.

126. Pedley RB, El-Emir E, Flynn AA, *et al.* (2002). Synergy between vascular targeting agents and antibody-directed therapy. *International Journal of Radiation Oncology, Biology, Physics* **54:** 1524–31.

127. Pedley RB, Boden JA, Boden R, *et al.* (1996). Ablation of colorectal xenografts with combined radioimmunotherapy and tumor blood flow-modifying agents. *Cancer Research* **15:** 3292–300.

128. Kinuya S, Yokoyama K, Koshida K, *et al.* (2004). Improved survival of mice bearing liver metastases of colon cancer cells treated with a combination of radioimmunotherapy and antiangiogenic therapy. *European Journal of Nuclear Medicine and Molecular Imaging* **31:** 981–5.

129. Blumenthal RD, Taylor A, Osorio L, *et al.* (2001). Optimizing the use of combined radioimmunotherapy and hypoxic cytotoxin therapy as a function of tumor hypoxia. *International Journal of Cancer* **94**: 564–71.

130. Meredith RF, Khazaeli MB, Plott WE, *et al.* (1996). Phase II study of dual ^{131}I-labelled monoclonal antibody therapy with interferon in patients with metastatic colorectal cancer. *Clinical Cancer Research* **2**: 1811–18.

131. Pallela VR, Rao SP, Thakur ML (2000). Interferon-alpha-2b immunoconjugate for improving immunoscintigraphy and immunotherapy. *Journal of Nuclear Medicine* **41**: 1108–13.

132. Greiner JW, Ullmann CD, Nieroda C, *et al.* (1993). Improved radioimmunotherapeutic efficacy of an anticarcinoma monoclonal antibody (^{131}I-CC49) when given in combination with gamma interferon. *Cancer Research* **53**: 600–8.

133. Behr TM, Sharkey RM, Sgouros G, *et al.* (1997). Overcoming the nephrotoxicity of radiometal-labelled immunoconjugates: improved cancer therapy administered to a mouse model in relation to the internal radiation dosimetry. *Cancer* **80**: 2591–610.

134. Behr TM, Sharkey RM, Juweid ME, *et al.* (1995). Reduction of the renal uptake of radiolabelled monoclonal antibody fragments by cationic amino acids and their derivatives. *Cancer Research* **55**: 3825–34.

135. Begent R, Keep PA, Green AJ, *et al.* (1982). Liposomally entrapped second antibody improves tumour imaging with radiolabelled (first) antitumour antibody. *Lancet* **ii**: 739–42.

136. Pedley RB, Dale R, Boden JA, Begent RHJ, Keep PA, Green AJ (1989). The effect of second antibody clearance on the distribution and dosimetry of radiolabelled anti-CEA antibody in a human colonic tumor xenograft model. *International Journal of Cancer* **43**: 713–18.

137. Goodwin DA, Mears CF, McTigue M, David GS (1986). Monoclonal antibody hapten radiopharmaceutical delivery. *Nuclear Medicine Communications* **7**: 569–80.

138. Goodwin DA, Mears CF, David GF, McTigue M, McCall MJ, Frincke JM, Stone MR (1986). Monoclonal antibodies as reversible equilibrium carriers of radiopharmaceuticals. *International Journal of Radiation Applications and Instrumentation B* **13**: 383–91.

139. Gruaz-Guyon A, Raguin O, Barbet J (2005). Recent advances in pretargeted radioimmunotherapy *Current Medicinal Chemistry* **12**: 319–338.

140. Langmuir VK, Mandonca HL (1992). The combined use of ^{131}I-labeled antibody and the hypoxic cytotoxin SR 4233 *in vitro* and *in vivo*. *Radiation Research* **132**: 351–8.

141. Goldenberg DM (2001). The role of radiolabelled antibodies in the treatment of non-Hodgkin's lymphoma: the coming of age of radioimmunotherapy. *Critical Reviews in Oncology/Hematology* **39**: 195–201.

142. Mulligan T, Carrasquillo JA, Chung Y, *et al.* (1995). Phase I study of intravenous Lu-labeled CC49 murine monoclonal antibody in patients with advanced adenocarcinoma. *Clinical Cancer Research* **1**: 1447–54.

143. Behr TM, Liersch T, Greiner-Bechert L, *et al.* (2002). Radioimmunotherapy of small-volume disease of metastatic colorectal cancer. *Cancer* **94**: 1373–81.

144. Tempero M, Keichner P, Dalrymple G, *et al.* (1997). High-dose therapy with iodine-131-labelled monoclonal antibody CC49 in patients with gastrointestinal cancers: a phase I trial. *Journal of Clinical Oncology* **15**: 1518–28.

145. Knox SJ, Goris ML, Tempero M, *et al.* (2000). Phase II trial of yttrium-90-DOTA-biotin pretargeted by NR-LU-10 antibody/streptavidin in patients with metastatic colon cancer. *Clinical Cancer Research* **6**: 406–14.

146. Buchegger F, Allal AS, Roth A, *et al.* (2000). Combined radioimmunotherapy and radiotherapy of liver metastases from colorectal cancer: a feasibility study. *Anticancer Research* **20**: 1889–96.

147. Meredith RF, Khazaeli MB, Lui T, *et al.* (1992). Dose fractionation of radiolabelled antibodies in oatients with metastatic colon cancer. *Journal of Nuclear Medicine* **33**: 1648–53.

148. DeNardo GL, Schlom J, Buchsbaum DJ *et al.* (2002). Rationales, evidence, and design considerations for fractionated radioimmunotherapy. *Cancer* **94**(4 Suppl), 1332–48.

149. Zeng Z-C, Tang ZY, Liu K-D, Xie H, Yao Z (1998). Improved long-term survival for unresectable hepatocellular carcinoma (HCC) with a combination of surgery and intrahepatic arterial infusion of ^{131}I-anti-HCC mAb. Phase I/II clinical trials. *Journal of Cancer Research and Clinical Oncology* **124**: 275–80.

150. Colcher D, Esteban J, Carrasquillo JA, *et al.* (1987). Complementation of intracavity and intravenous administration of a monoclonal antibody (B72.3) in patients with carcinoma. *Cancer Research* **47**: 4218–24.

151. Wong JYC, Shibata S, Williams LE, *et al.* (2003). A phase I trial of ^{90}Y-anti-carcinoembryonic antigen chimeric T84.66 radioimmunotherapy with 5-fluorouracil in patients with metastatic colorectal cancer. *Clinical Cancer Research* **9**: 5842–52.

152. Burger PC, Heinz ER, Shibata T, Kleihues P (1988). Topographic anatomy and CT correlations in the untreated glioblastoma multiforme. *Journal of Neurosurgery* **68**: 698–704.

153. Wallner KE, Galicich JH, Krol G, Arbit E, Malkin MG (1989). Patterns of failure following treatment for glioblastoma multiforme and anaplastic astrocytoma. *International Journal of Radiation Oncology, Biology, Physics* **16**: 1405–9.

154. Riva P, Franceschi G, Arista A, *et al.* (1997). Local application of radiolabelled monoclonal antibodies in the treatment of high grade malignant gliomas: a six year clinical experience. *Cancer* **80**: 2733–42.

155. Kalafonos HP, Pawlikowska TR, Hemingway A, *et al.* (1989). Antibody guided diagnosis and therapy of brain gliomas using radiolabelled monoclonal antibodies against epidermal growth factor receptor and placental alkaline phosphatase. *Journal of Nuclear Medicine* **30**: 1636–45.

156. Zalutsky MR, Cheung NK, Humm JL, *et al.* (1990). Monoclonal antibody and F(ab')$_2$ fragment delivery to tumor in patients with glioma: comparison of intracarotid and intravenous administration. *Cancer Research.* **50**: 4105–10.

157. Brown MT, Coleman RE, Friedman AH, *et al.* (1996). Intrathecal ^{131}I-labeled antitenascin monoclonal antibody 81C6 treatment of patients with leptomeningeal neoplasms or primary brain tumor resection cavities with subarachnoid communication: phase I trials results. *Clinical Cancer Research* **2**: 963–72.

158. Riva P, Arista A, Franceschi G, *et al.* (1995). Local treatment of malignant gliomas by direct infusion of specific monoclonal antibodies labelled with [131]I: comparison of the results obtained in recurrent and newly diagnosed tumours. *Cancer Research.* **55**: 5952–6s.

159. Paganelli G, Bartolomei M, Ferrari M, *et al.* (2001). Pre-targeted locoregional radioimmunotherapy with ^{90}Y-biotin in glioma patients: phase I study and

preliminary therapeutic results. *Cancer Biotherapy and Radiopharmaceuticals* **16**: 227–35.

160. Bartolomei M, Mazzetta C, Handkiewicz-Junak D, *et al.* (2004). Combined treatment of glioblastoma patients with locoregional pre-targeted ^{90}Y-biotin radioimmunotherapy and temozolomide. *Quarterly Journal of Nuclear Medicine* **48**: 220–8.

Suggested reading

Begent RHJ, Pedley RB (1990). Antibody targeted therapy in cancer: Comparison of murine and clinical studies. *Cancer Treatment Reviews* **17**: 373–8.

Chester K, Pedley B, Tolner *et al.* (2004). Engineering antibodies for clinical applications in cancer. *Tumor Biology* **25**: 91–8.

Goldenberg DM (2003). Advancing the role of radiolabeled antibodies in the therapy of cancer. *Cancer Immunology and Immunotherapy* **52**: 281–96.

Hagenbeek A (2005). Future trends in radioimmunotherapy. *Seminars in Oncology* **32**: S57–62.

Holliger P, Hudson PJ (2005). Engineered antibody fragments and the rise of single domains. *Nature Biotechnology* **23**: 1126–36.

Huhalov A, Chester KA (2004). Engineered single chain antibody fragments for radioimmunotherapy. *Quarterly Journal of Nuclear Medicine and Molecular Imaging* **48**: 279–88.

Koppe MJ, Bleichrodt RP, Oyen WJG, Boerman OC (2005). Radioimmunotherapy and colorectal cancer. *British Journal of Surgery* **92**: 264–76.

Larson SM, Krenning EP (2005). A pragmatic perspective on molecular targeted radionuclide therapy. *Journal of Nuclear Medicine* **46**: 1–3S.

Mather SJ, Britton KE (2004). Radioimmunotherapy. Progress, potential and problems. *Quarterly Journal of Nuclear Medicine and Molecular Imaging* **48**: 248–50.

von Mehren M, Adams GP, Weiner LM (2003). Monoclonal antibody therapy for cancer. *Annual Review of Medicine* **54**: 343–69.

Napier MP, Begent RHJ (1998). Radioimmunotherapy of gastrointestinal cancer. In: Riva T (ed.), *Cancer radioimmunotherapy*, pp. 333–88. Boston: Harwood Academia.

Pedley RB (1996). Pharmacokinetics of monoclonal antibodies. Implications for their use in cancer therapy. *Clinical Immunotherapy* **6**: 54–67.

Sharkey RM, Goldenberg DM (2005). Perspectives on cancer therapy with radiolabeled monoclonal antibodies. *Journal of Nuclear Medicine* **46**: 115–27S.

Zalutsky MR (2005). Current status of therapy of solid tumors: brain tumor therapy. *Journal of Nuclear Medicine* **46**: 151–6S.

Chapter 3

Radiotherapy for benign thyroid disease: use of ^{131}I

Steve Hyer, Clive Harmer

3.1 Background to use

Radioactive iodine began being employed for the treatment of hyperthyroidism in the 1940s when it first became possible to extract large quantities of the isotope ^{131}I with a half-life of 8 days. Prior to this, only very short-lived isotopes such as ^{128}I (half-life of 25 minutes) or ^{130}I (half-life 12.5 hours) could be extracted and these were too short-lived to be useful as therapy[1]. Initially it was used in the elderly or those unfit for surgery because of concern about its potential carcinogenic effects.

The fear of carcinogenic effects of radioiodine receded as long-term studies reported no special risk. The Co-operative Thyrotoxicosis Therapy Follow-up Study published in 1974 reported a fivefold increased incidence of thyroid carcinoma in adults with Graves' disease treated medically with thionamides compared with those treated with ^{131}I and an eightfold increase versus those treated surgically[2]. These observations over 10–20 years of follow-up suggested that an increased risk of thyroid malignancy could be related to the persistence of thyroid tissue in patients treated with drugs compared with those receiving radioiodine or surgery. The alternative explanation that the medication was carcinogenic seems unlikely. There was no evidence of an excess of thyroid cancer in adults following ^{131}I therapy. Similarly, no evidence emerged of an increase in leukaemia[3] or solid tumours in patients receiving radioiodine, with the possible exception of gastric carcinoma in one report[4].

With more than 50 years experience, radioiodine has become a popular treatment for hyperthyroidism due to either Graves' disease or nodular goitre (solitary adenoma or multinodular goitre).

This chapter will review the place of radioiodine in the therapy of patients with benign toxic and non-toxic thyroid disease. There is no place for radioiodine in the treatment of inflammatory thyroid disorders.

3.2 **Clinical indications**

Radioiodine (^{131}I) therapy is indicated in the treatment of hyperthyroidism due to Graves' disease or toxic nodular goitre (solitary adenoma or multinodular goitre). It is also indicated when hyperthyroidism recurs after thyroid surgery, or for persistent hyperthyroidism after previous [131]I. In addition, radioiodine is used successfully to reduce the size of large non-toxic multinodular goitres.

Treatment with ^{131}I is contraindicated in thyrotoxicosis due to thyroiditis or to iodine excess (such as occurs with amiodarone therapy) as in these conditions there is little or no iodine uptake by the thyroid gland.

In the UK, radioiodine is generally given to patients with Graves' disease whose hyperthyroidism relapses after a course of antithyroid drug treatment, although some clinicians prescribe radioiodine as first-line therapy[5]. Another group of patients with Graves' disease eligible for ^{131}I are those who develop serious adverse effects from antithyroid medication such as agranulocytosis.

Radioiodine may be safely given to patients of all age groups but is less often given to children less than 10 years old with Graves' disease as described later.

Radioiodine is the treatment of choice for toxic nodular goitre[6]. Most patients experience some reduction in the goitre size after ^{131}I therapy. This observation has been extended to patients with large non-toxic diffuse goitres[7]. A reduction in non-toxic goitre size of about 50% has been reported within 12–18 months[7]. In nodular goitre, pretreatment with low-dose recombinant human thyroid-stimulating hormone (TSH) may result in a greater reduction in goitre size relative to the administered dose of radioiodine[8].

3.3 **Typical doses**

There are very wide variations in clinical practice for the treatment of thyrotoxicosis, with some clinicians preferring an ablative dose of radioiodine while others use smaller doses. Ablative therapy has the advantage of quicker resolution of the hyperthyroidism thereby minimizing potential morbidity such as cardiac arrhythmia. Smaller doses, based on calculation of the precise dose of radioactivity absorbed by the thyroid, potentially minimize the incidence of subsequent hypothyroidism.

There is no consensus regarding the ideal first dose of radioiodine in the treatment of hyperthyroidism[9]. Some investigators recommend a calculated [131]iodine activity in the range of 200 Gy[10]. Others prefer a fixed dose regimen. Doses ranging from 5 to 10 mCi (185–370 MBq) have previously been recommended[11,12]. A recent Finnish study[13] concluded that the remission rate after a fixed dose of 7 mCi (259 MBq) in hyperthyroidism was not significantly different from the larger 10 mCi fixed dose and advocated this as the first empirical dose.

Table 3.1 Recommended radioiodine activity in hyperthyroidism[6]

Indication	Clinical details	Guide activity
First presentation Graves' disease	Moderate goitre (40–50 g) No significant eye signs*	400–550 MBq
Toxic multinodular goitre	Older person, mild heart failure Atrial fibrillation or other co-morbidity (e.g. cancer)†	At least 550 MBq
Toxic adenoma	Mild hyperthyroidism usually	300–500 MBq

*If associated significant thyroid eye disease, options are to postpone radioiodine treatment until eye problems have become stable, proceed with radioiodine with careful thyroid monitoring avoiding thyroid dysfunction, or administration of glucocorticoids with radioiodine and continued for further 4 weeks.

†In patients with severe accompanying co-morbidity, ablative therapy up to 800 MBq may be administered as an outpatient. Hospitalization is required if a greater activity is used.

The Royal College of Physicians Guidelines (1995) offers guidance based on the aetiology of the hyperthyroidism and any co-morbidity (Table 3.1). The Guidelines state that although an ablative strategy may be more cost-effective than smaller doses, consideration should be given to the health gain value of remaining euthyroid. There is general agreement that the period of hyperthyroidism should be minimized in the elderly because of their greater risk of adverse cardiovascular effects, such that in this group of patients a larger dose of radioiodine is justified.

Retrospective analysis of patients with Graves' disease at the Royal Marsden Hospital had suggested that an absorbed dose of 60 Gy to the thyroid would be optimal to achieve euthyroidism[14]; a similar conclusion was reached more recently[15]. Using this dose, results from our Unit at 5 years are encouraging, although a dose of 120 Gy is needed for patients with a large thyroid volume (>30 ml) and for patients with a micronodular thyroids demonstrated by ultrasound[16,17]. A suggested pathway of treatment as used in our department is shown in Appendix 3.1.

The influence of antithyroid drugs on the outcome of ^{131}I therapy for hyperthyroidism is controversial. These agents, particularly propylthiouracil, appear to render the thyroid gland relatively resistant to radioiodine and hence it is recommended that they are stopped for at least 2 days prior to ^{131}I therapy[6]. There is evidence that patients maintained on antithyroid drugs for many years before being treated with radioiodine become radioresistant, thus requiring doses of 400 MBq (11 mCi) or more[18].

3.4 **Precautions and side-effects in use**

The administration of radioiodine is tightly regulated by the Administration of Radioactive Substances Advisory Committee (ARSAC) and by the Protection Of Persons Undergoing Medical Examination or Treatment (POPUMET) regulations[6]. Only medical staff holding an appropriate ARSAC certificate may authorize its administration. Certificates are granted to individuals who can demonstrate adequate training, experience, and competence in the administration of radioactive substances. Disposal of urine is considered safe when passed down the lavatory. Patients with urinary incontinence are not suitable for radioiodine treatment. The number of days for which patients need to take special precautions regarding contact with others is shown in Table 3.2.

Radioiodine treatment is absolutely contraindicated in pregnancy and during lactation as ^{131}I can cross the placenta into the developing fetus or be passed via breast milk into the baby. No patient in whom there is a possibility of being pregnant should receive radioiodine. Similarly, breast feeding cannot continue once radioiodine has been administered.

If necessary a pregnancy test can be performed to confirm that the patient is not pregnant at the time of radioiodine administration. Thyroid development begins at about the 12th week of gestation. Therapeutic administration of radioiodine to the mother will usually result in fetal hypothyroidism and may be associated with attention-deficit disorders or memory impairment in the offspring in later life[19].

Table 3.2 Number of days for which patients should take special precautions according to the activity of radioiodine administered[6]

	Administered activity ^{131}I (MBq)			
Precaution	**200**	**400**	**600**	**800**
Avoid journeys on public transport	0	0	1	2
Stay off work (even when it does not involve close contact with other people)	0	0	1	2
Avoid places of entertainment or close contact with other people	1	5	9	12
Stay off work (when it involves close contact with other people)	1	5	9	12
Avoid non-essential close personal contact with children and with pregnant women; work that involves close contact with children; radiosensitive work	14	21	24	27

Patient may travel home by private transport for administered activities greater than 400 MBq but not more than 800 MBq. Total close contact time with any individual should not exceed 1 hour.

The hazard to a fetus from exposure to a family member, not the mother, who has been treated with radioiodine is extremely small and can be minimized by adherence to standard post-treatment guidelines (Table 3.2). Women are advised not to become pregnant for 4 months after receiving radioiodine. If pregnancy does occur sooner than 4 months after administration, advice should be sought but termination is not mandatory[6]. Male patients should similarly avoid fathering a child for 4 months after ^{131}I administration.

Thyroid cancer has been reported in a few children who had received radioiodine for thyrotoxicosis and there is also an increased risk of benign thyroid nodules following this treatment[2,20]. The increase in thyroid cancers in children followed massive radioiodine exposure after the Chernobyl disaster is well documented[21]. These observations have made clinicians managing childhood Graves' disease wary of using ^{131}I therapy. However, a recent study with nearly 40 years of follow-up data showed no increased risk of thyroid cancer or leukaemia in children and adolescents treated with radioiodine[22]. The reports of increased risk of cancer or thyroid nodules occurred in children receiving only low-dose [131]I (<75 mCi/g thyroid tissue). It is recommended that when treating children the dose selected should achieve thyroid destruction[23].

Controversy persists regarding potential worsening of thyroid eye disease after radioiodine treatment[24]. A large US study showed that if there is no thyroid eye disease at the time of treatment with ^{131}I, the chance of it developing was low and comparable with carbimazole treatment or thyroid surgery[25].

Subsequent studies from Italy[26] and Sweden[27] demonstrated that patients with significant thyroid eye disease prior to radioiodine show definite deterioration of this condition after radioiodine administration. In the Italian study, nine of 26 patients (35%) with pre-existing thyroid eye disease showed progression after ^{131}I therapy, but this did not occur in patients concomitantly given glucocorticoids. In the Swedish study, thyroid eye disease either developed or progressed in 10% of methimazole-treated patients, 16% of those submitted to thyroidectomy and 33% of ^{131}I-treated patients ($P = 0.02$ versus other treatments).

Bartalena and colleagues[28] went on to show that treatment with corticosteroids could prevent deterioration of the eyes after radioiodine. In this prospective randomized controlled study of 450 patients with Graves' thyrotoxicosis, thyroid eye disease worsened in 23 of 150 radioiodine-treated patients (15%) but in only 3% of methimazole-treated patients; radioiodine-associated progression of thyroid eye disease was prevented by a short course of corticosteroids. The study used 0.4–0.5 mg prednisolone/kg body weight starting 2–3 days after ^{131}I and continuing for 3 months (tapering off over the last 2 months). Risk factors for progression of eye disease after ^{131}I therapy in that study were pre-existing thyroid ophthalmopathy, cigarette smoking, severe hyperthyroidism, late correction of post-radioiodine hypothyroidism, and high TSH-receptor antibody titres. Early administration of thyroxine to prevent hypothyroidism can reduce the risk of Graves' ophthalmopathy after radioiodine[29].

The consensus view appears to be that for patients with no sign of thyroid eye disease at the time of radioiodine administration, ^{131}I therapy is safe and effective. For patients with signs of Graves' ophthalmopathy, radioiodine may exacerbate the eye disease. The options are to avoid radioiodine altogether, particularly in high-risk patients (smokers or those with severe hyperthyroidism), or to give concomitant prednisolone for 3 months. Early replacement with thyroxine should be considered for these patients. It should be noted that although studies have shown transient worsening of thyroid eye disease after ^{131}I, there is little evidence of long-term adverse effects.

Another area of controversy is transient worsening of hyperthyroidism in the first 2 weeks following radioiodine, potentially severe enough to cause a 'thyroid storm.' This has been ascribed to ^{131}I-induced thyroiditis and release of stored thyroxine. Case reports have appeared in the literature from time to time[30], but it is not clear whether withdrawal of antithyroid medication prior to giving radioiodine may be responsible rather than the radioiodine[31]; this may be particularly the case in children. Both the duration of stopping antithyroid medication prior to radioiodine and the dose of ^{131}I administered may be relevant[31].

Because of the risk of transient hyperthyroidism, the Royal College of Physicians[6] recommends warning patients of the possibility of experiencing palpitations or other hyperthyroid symptoms, especially if not euthyroid prior to ^{131}I therapy. Furthermore, elderly patients and those with heart failure may be particularly at risk and in these patients a period of observation in hospital may be indicated. In our experience, this complication is very rare when using doses of 400 MBq or less.

Antithyroid medication to deplete the thyroid of thyroxine is also recommended in the at-risk elderly patient so as to achieve euthyroidism prior to treatment. Antithyroid medication may be restarted 3 days after ^{131}I treatment.

3.5 Practical considerations

Radioiodine must be prescribed by an ARSAC license holder. The individual dose may be ordered as a unit dose from the supplier or dispensed from a local stock solution. Capsules are usually obtained within 72 hours of administration but liquid formulations may require more than 1 week's notice. Individual patient doses must be measured in the medical physics department prior to administration to ensure that the activity is within 10% of the dose prescribed. Capsules are generally preferred to liquid preparations and are safer for staff. They dissolve readily in warm or hot water and it is usual practice for patients to have a hot drink (e.g. tea) after dose administration. Liquid formulations have a greater hazard of spill compared with capsules. Patients with dentures should remove these prior to administration to prevent ^{131}I being trapped under the dental plate. After administration, patients should rinse and swallow water.

Prior to administration, the nurse should confirm that the patient has given signed consent for the treatment, is not pregnant or breast-feeding, has stopped antithyroid medication for at least 3 days and has received and read information regarding any restrictions following the treatment. Restrictions will depend on the activity given, the home, work, and travel arrangements. Patients are told to avoid pregnancy for at least 4 months. The importance of attending follow-up appointments is emphasized with blood tests for thyroid function performed shortly before each clinic visit.

3.6 **Clinical efficacy**

There have been few randomized clinical trials to compare the efficacy of different doses of ^{131}I in the treatment of hyperthyroidism. The earliest compared a conventional dose of 5.18 MBq/g adjusted for thyroid size by palpation with half this dose in 546 patients with various causes of thyrotoxicosis[32]. Although initial control of hyperthyroidism was slower in the low-dose group, results at 3 years were very similar.

A second trial[10] compared a standard activity of 555 MBq ^{131}I with an activity calculated to deliver 100 Gy, based on thyroid ultrasound and radioiodine kinetics. Success at 6 months with the elimination of hyperthyroidism was 71% for the fixed activity vs. 58% adjusted activity; higher success rates were found in small volume thyroids. More recently Leslie et al.[33] reported similar rates of hypothyroidism and persistent hyperthyroidism in patients assigned to either fixed doses (235–350 MBq) or adjusted doses (2.96 MBq/g or 4.44 MBq/g thyroid). Very few patients (6.8%) achieved euthyroidism by the end of the study (median follow-up 80 months): nearly a quarter of patients were hyperthyroid and about 70% hypothyroid.

The definition of success in assessing treatment of hyperthyroidism by radioactive iodine is controversial. Most investigators consider hyperthyroidism 'cured' if sufficient thyroid tissue has been destroyed to render the patient *either* euthyroid *or* hypothyroid[12]. Using this definition, a cure rate approaching 100% is achievable after one or more treatments[34].

Most studies show the predicted dose–response relationship between administered radioactivity and rate of hypothyroidism. Using a single administration of 370 MBq in patients with hyperthyroidism due to either Graves' disease or toxic nodular goitre, Allahabadia et al.[12] reported a cure rate of 84.6%, with 60.8% becoming hypothyroid by 1 year.

An alternative and stricter view is to consider only achievement of the euthyroid state after radioiodine as success. The problem with this approach is that hypothyroidism may arise many years after therapy and indeed may be inevitable in the long-term. An annual incidence of 2–3% of hypothyroidism is commonly observed even after low-dose therapy[12]. A further problem is the definition of euthyroidism, as a suppressed TSH may persist for years after treatment in clinically euthyroid patients[35].

Nevertheless, a more conservative approach aiming to achieve a euthyroid state and delay hypothyroidism may be a reasonable approach in a patients with a small thyroid mass and perhaps also in younger patients. Low-dose [131]I (74 MBq or 2 mCi) given at 6-monthly intervals achieved euthyroidism in 46% of patients with Graves' disease at 12 months and 75% at the end of 2 years with a yearly incidence of hypothyroidism of only 4–6%[36]. With longer follow-up, the same group found a 20% incidence of hypothyroidism at 6 years[37]. More recently, doses of 90 Gy were reported to achieve euthyroidism in 46% of patients with a median follow-up of 37.5 (24–48) months[15]; 47% of patients were rendered hypothyroid and 7% remained hyperthyroid at the end of the observation period.

We recently reported 84 patients with either Graves' disease (52), Graves' in a nodular goitre (13), or toxic nodular goitre (19) who had been treated with 60 Gy ^{131}I and with complete follow-up data[17]. At 5 years, 40 (48%) patients were euthyroid defined as normal thyroid function for a minimum of 3 years on no thyroid medication. A total of 34 (40%) had become hypothyroid requiring thyroxine, 10 within 6 months of treatment. The remaining 10 patients were euthyroid (<3 years) following further doses of radioiodine. Patients with larger than average thyroid volumes (>30 ml), patients with a clinically nodular thyroid and those who had received >24 months antithyroid medication prior to radioiodine were more likely to relapse and require further treatment. Thus nearly half of all patients treated with 60 Gy radioiodine achieved stable euthyroidism at 5 years. A larger initial dose seems warranted in patients with high-risk factors for relapse. Low-dose treatment appears to minimize early hypothyroidism but patients will need to continue antithyroid medication longer until euthyroidism is achieved. We advocate a second dose of ^{131}I if the patient remains hyperthyroid (on medication) 12 months after initial treatment.

Several studies have indicated that the major factors determining poor response to radioiodine are severe hyperthyroidism at diagnosis, male gender, and large thyroid volumes[11,38]. These factors should be taken into account when planning treatment: patients with large goitres, very high serum-free thyroxine at diagnosis, especially if male, should receive higher ^{131}I doses.

Retrospective data on the long-term risk of hypothyroidism after radio-iodine for patients with Graves' disease suggest that hypothyroidism seems almost inevitable. Thus by 36 years, all but two of 116 patients with Graves' disease had become hypothyroid after doses of 5–6 mCi[22]. In another long-term study, hypothyroidism developed in 82% of Graves' patients treated with 7 mCi (259 MBq) [131]I by 25 years[13].

Results of radioiodine treatment for toxic multinodular goitre are similar to those for Graves' patients. Cure rates (defined as hypothyroidism or euthyroidism) of about 70% are reported[12,13], although the incidence of hypothyroidism is lower compared with Graves' disease[13]. This might relate to preferential uptake of radioiodine by the hyperfunctioning nodules leaving normal thyroid tissue relatively unaffected. With a solitary toxic nodule, euthyroidism is commonly achieved after a dose of about 20 mCi[8].

The use of ^{131}I therapy for the reduction in size of non-toxic goitres is controversial. While guidelines exist for the evaluation and treatment of hyperthyroidism and hypothyroidism, there is no consensus on the use of radioiodine in euthyroid patients with a large goitre. While surgery remains the treatment of choice for patients with large goitres and obstructive symptoms, radioiodine may be an option in patients unfit or unwilling to undergo operative treatment.

In a recent review of published studies, Bonnema and colleagues[18] concluded that radioiodine treatment has a favourable effect on tracheal compression and inspiratory capacity but the reduction in thyroid volume is only 30–40% within about 2 years.

Many studies can be criticized as not having a control group and there is debate regarding thyroid volume assessment, with most studies reporting great individual variation in response.

Treatment of large goitres typically involves high-dose ^{131}I activity. A median dose of 2281 MBq or 61.6 mCi (range, 988–4620 MBq or 26.7–124.9 mCi) was used in a typical study[39]. Unless this treatment is fractionated, patients need hospitalization. Prior administration of low-dose recombinant human TSH can double ^{131}I uptake and initial results in patients with large non-toxic multinodular goitres are promising[8].

One concern is that high-dose radioiodine could induce thyroid oedema in these patients aggravating airways obstruction. Indeed, in one study[39], a 15%

increase in goitre size was observed in the first week of treatment in a group of euthyroid and hyperthyroid patients with very large goitres. Although not universally reported, unexpected worsening of obstruction shortly after treatment should be anticipated and consideration given to glucocorticoid treatment to reduce inflammatory oedema. Estimation of the smallest tracheal cross-sectional area by MRI is a useful guide for airways obstruction and correlates with inspiratory capacity in very large goitres[39]. The 1-year risk of hypothyroidism after treatment of large goitres is estimated to be 14–22%[18], such that all patients need regular follow-up.

3.7 Alternative treatments and relative role/efficacy of [131]I

Thyroidectomy was frequently performed in the past for Graves' disease. In competent hands, the risk of hypoparathyroidism or recurrent laryngeal nerve damage is less than 1% With the advent of more effective medical treatments, surgical treatment has become less popular unless coexistent thyroid cancer is suspected. Surgery also remains the preferred treatment for patients with a large or retrosternal goitre causing obstructive symptoms[18].

The optimal extent of thyroidectomy (subtotal or near-total) remains controversial, although there is a move towards near-total thyroidectomy in order to reduce the incidence of recurrent thyrotoxicosis. Surgery is an alternative to radioiodine where prolonged antithyroid medication has failed and for patients developing a reaction to the drugs such as agranulocytosis. In patients with severe thyroid eye disease, treatment with antithyroid drugs followed by thyroidectomy is an alternative to use of ^{131}I and may be less likely to exacerbate ophthalmopathy[40].

In long-term follow-up following surgery, recurrence of goitre is surprisingly high, of the order of 15–40%, especially in nodular goitres[41], although can be reduced by administration of thyroxine. Even when patients are clinically euthyroid, subtle abnormalities of thyroid function can frequently be demonstrated following subtotal thyroidectomy by thyrotrophin-releasing hormone-stimulation testing[42]. After 10 years and depending on the extent of the original surgery, 20–40% of patients are hypothyroid[43].

In the past, enthusiastic surgeons have recommended surgery for all children as initial treatment, claiming that there was less interference with normal growth and development than with prolonged antithyroid drug treatment. The advantage of antithyroid medication is that it avoids the psychological and physical problems caused by surgery in this age group. With drugs the need for surgery (or ^{131}I) can be delayed until conditions become favourable[44].

Surgery inevitably leaves a permanent scar that can be cosmetically unattractive, especially in young females. The recurrence rate is higher by up to 15% in children compared with that observed in adults. There is always a small risk of permanent hypothyroidism and damage to the recurrent laryngeal nerves. Hypoparathyroidism necessitates a complicated medical programme that may be life-long, and is the major reason for opposing routine surgical therapy in this disease.

Surgery is relatively contraindicated in patients with coincident severe heart or lung disease. It is technically difficult and more hazardous to perform in patients who have undergone previous thyroid surgery. Surgery is not recommended during the first or third trimesters of pregnancy as it may induce abortion or premature labour, respectively. Only surgeons trained and experienced in thyroid surgery should undertake thyroidectomy[45]. It should also be noted that the cost of radioiodine therapy is substantially less than surgical treatment, which usually requires a 3–5-day stay in hospital[6].

Thyroxine has been used for many years in an attempt to reduce goitre size in both diffuse and nodular thyroid enlargement. Evidence for its efficacy is limited, especially with large goitres. In a randomized trial comparing thyroxine with radioiodine, thyroxine was found to have no significant effect on goitre size over 2 years and was associated with significant bone loss[46].

3.8 Concluding remarks

Although used routinely for over 50 years, many aspects of radioiodine treatment in benign thyroid disease are controversial owing to the lack of large prospective randomized studies comparing efficacy, side-effects, cost, and patient satisfaction. Nevertheless, ^{131}I is devoid of major side-effects and can be used safely for patients with Graves' disease or toxic multinodular goitre. It is the treatment of choice for a solitary autonomous toxic nodule. There is increasing interest in its use for patients with large non-toxic goitre, particularly if patients are unsuitable or unwilling to undergo surgery.

References

1. Hertz S, Roberts A (1942). Application of radioactive iodine in therapy of Graves' disease. *Journal of Clinical Investigation* **21**: 624–6.
2. Dobyns BM, Sheline GE, Workman JB, *et al.* (1974). Malignant and benign neoplasms of the thyroid in patients treated for hyperthyroidism: a report of the co-operative thyrotoxicosis therapy follow-up study. *Journal of Clinical Endocrinology and Metabolism* **38**: 976–98.
3. Hall P, Boice JD, Berg G, *et al.* (1992). Leukaemia incidence after iodine-131 exposure. *Lancet* **340**: 1–4.

4. Holm LE, Hall P, Wiklund K, *et al.* (1991). Cancer risk after iodine-131 therapy for hyperthyroidism. *Journal of the National Cancer Institute* **83**: 1072–7.

5. Hedley AJ, Lazarus JH, McGhee SM, *et al.* (1992). Treatment of hyperthyroidism by radioactive iodine. Summary of a UK National Survey prepared for the Royal College of Physicians Committee on Endocrinology and Diabetes. *Journal of the Royal College of Physicians London* **26**: 348–51.

6. Royal College of Physicians (1995). *Guidelines for the use of radioiodine in the management of hyperthyroidism*. London: Royal College of Physicians.

7. Nygaard B, Faber J, Veje A, Hansen JEM (1997). Thyroid volume and function after 131I treatment of diffuse non-toxic goitre. *Clinical Endocrinology* **46**: 493–6.

8. Huysmans DA, Nieuwlaat W-A, Hermus AR (2004). Towards larger volume reduction of nodular goitres by radioiodine therapy: a role for pre-treatment with recombinant human thyrotropin? *Clinical Endocrinology* **60**: 297–9.

9. Kalinyak JE, McDougall IR (2003). How should the dose of iodine-131 be determined in the treatment of Graves' hyperthyroidism? *Journal of Clinical Endocrinology and Metabolism* **88**: 975–7.

10. Peters H, Fischer C, Bogner U, *et al.* (1995). Radioiodine therapy of Graves' hyperthyroidism: standard vs. calculated 131iodine activity. Results from a prospective randomised multicentre study. *European Journal of Clinical Investigation* **25**: 186–93.

11. Watson AB, Brownie BE, Frampton CM, *et al.* (1988). Outcome following a standardised 185 MBq dose 131I therapy for Graves' disease. *Clinical Endocrinology* **28**: 487–96.

12. Allahabadia A, Daykin J, Sheppard MC, *et al.* (2001). Radioiodine treatment of hyperthyroidism—prognostic factors for outcome. *Journal of Clinical Endocrinology and Metabolism* **86**: 3611–17.

13. Metso S, Jaatinen P, Huhtala H, *et al.* (2004). Long term follow-up study of radioiodine treatment of hyperthyroidism. *Clinical Endocrinology* **61**: 641–8.

14. Flower M, Al-Saadi A, Harmer CL, McCready VR, Ott RJ (1994). Dose-response study on thyrotoxic patients undergoing positron emission tomography and radioiodine therapy. *European Journal of Nuclear Medicine* **21**: 531–6.

15. Howarth D, Epstein M, Lan L, *et al.* (2001). Determination of the optimum minimum radioiodine dose in patients with Graves' disease: a clinical outcome study. *European Journal of Nuclear Medicine* **28**: 1489–95.

16. Hyer SL, Pratt BE, McCready VR, Flower MA, Harmer CL (2001). Clinical outcome of patients with Graves' disease treated with a single absorbed dose of 60 Gy to the thyroid. *European Federation of Endocrine Societies Abstracts* 865.

17. Hyer SL, Pratt BE, Haq M, Harmer CL (2004). Clinical outcome at 5 years in patients with thyrotoxicosis treated with low dose radioiodine. *Abstracts of 12th International Congress of Endocrinology* 644.

18. Bonnema SJ, Bartalena L, Toft AD, Hegedus L (2002). Controversies in radioiodine therapy: relation to ophthalmopathy, the possible radioprotective effect of antithyroid drugs and use in large goitres. *European Journal of Endocrinology* **147**: 1–11.

19. Gorman CA (1999). Radioiodine and pregnancy. *Thyroid* **9**: 721–6.

20. Rivkees SA, Sklar C, Freemark M (1998). Clinical review 99: the management of Graves disease in children with special emphasis on radioiodine treatment. *Journal of Clinicial Endocrinology and Metabolism* **83**: 3767–76.

21. Tuttle RM, Becker DV (2000). The Chernobyl accident and its consequences: update at the millennium. *Seminars in Nuclear Medicine* **30**: 133–40.

22. Read CH, Tansey MJ, Menda Y (2004). A 36-year retrospective analysis of the efficacy and safety of radioactive iodine in treating young Graves' patients. *Journal of Clinical Endocrinology and Metabolism* **89**: 4229–4233.

23. Rivkees S (2004). Radioactive iodine use in childhood Graves disease: time to wake up and smell the I-131. *Journal of Clinical Endocrinology and Metabolism* **89**: 4227–8.

24. Noury AMS, Stanford MR, Graham EM (2001). Radioiodine and Graves ophthalmopathy reconsidered. *Nuclear Medicine Communications* **22**: 1167–9.

25. Sridama V, DeGroot LJ (1989). Treatment of Graves' disease and the course of opthalmopathy. *American Journal of Medicine* **87**: 70–3.

26. Bartalena L, Marcocci C, Bogazzi F, *et al.* (1989). Use of corticosteroids to prevent progression of Graves' ophthalmopathy after radioiodine therapy for hyperthyroidism. *New England Journal of Medicine* **321**: 1349–52.

27. Tallstedt L, Lundell G, Torring O (1992). Occurrence of ophthalmopathy after treatment for Graves' hyperthyroidism. *New England Journal of Medicine* **362**: 1733–8.

28. Bartalena L, Marocci C, Bogazzi F, *et al.* (1998). Relation between therapy for hyperthyroidism and the course of Graves' ophthalmopathy. *New England Journal of Medicine* **338**: 73–8.

29. Tallstedt L, Lundell G, Blomgren H (1994). Does early administration of thyroxine reduce the development of Graves' ophthalmopathy after radioactive treatment. *European Journal of Endocrinology* **130**: 494–7.

30. McDermott MT, Kidd GS, Dodson LE Jr, Hofeldt FD (1983). Radioiodine-induced thyroid storm. Case report and literature review. *American Journal of Medicine* **75**: 353–9.

31. Kadmon PM, Noto RB, Boney CM, Goodwin G, Gruppuso PA (2001). Thyroid storm in a child following radioactive iodine (RAI) therapy: a consequence of RAI *versus* withdrawal of antithyroid medication. *Journal of Clinical Endocrinology and Metabolism* **86**: 1865–67.

32. Smith RN, Wilson GM (1967). Clinical trial of different doses of 131I in treatment of thyrotoxicosis. *British Medical Journal* **21**: 129–32.

33. Leslie WD, Ward L, Salamon EA, *et al.* (2003). A randomised comparison of radioiodine doses in Graves' hyperthyroidism. *Journal of Clinical Endocrinology and Metabolism* **88**: 978–83.

34. Franklyn JA, Daykin J, Droic Z, *et al.* (1991). Long-term follow-up of treatment of thyrotoxicosis by three different methods. *Clinical Endocrinology* **34**: 71–6.

35. Davies PH, Franklyn JA, Daykin J, Sheppard MC (1992). The significance of TSH values measured in a sensitive assay in the follow-up of hyperthyroid patients treated with radioiodine. *Journal of Clinical Endocrinology and Metabolism* **74**: 1189–1194.

36. Hoskin PJ, Spathis GS, McCready VR, Cosgrove DO, Harmer CL (1985). Low-dose radioiodine given six-monthly in Graves' disease. *Journal of the Royal Society of Medicine* **78**: 893–5.

37. Lowdell CP, Dobbs HJ, Spathis GS, McCready VR, Cosgrove DO, Harmer CL (1985). Low dose ^{131}I in treatment of Graves' disease. *Journal of the Royal Society of Medicine* **78**: 197–202.

38. Nordyke RA, Gilbert FI (1991). Optimal iodine-131 dose for eliminating hyperthyroidism in Graves' disease. *Journal of Nuclear Medicine* **32**: 411–16.

39. Bonnema SJ, Bertelsen H, Mortensen J, *et al.* (1999). The feasibility of high dose iodine 131 treatment as an alternative to surgery in patients with a very large goiter: effect on thyroid function and size and pulmonary function. *Journal of Clinical Endocrinology and Metabolism* **84**: 3636–41.

40. Torring O, Tallstedt L, Wallin G, *et al.* (1996). Graves' hyperthyroidism: Treatment with antithyroid drugs, surgery, or radioiodine-a prospective, randomized study. *Journal of Clinical Endocrinology and Metabolism* **81**: 2986–93.

41. Roejdmark J, Jaerhult J (1995). High long term recurrence rate after subtotal thyroidectomy for nodular goitre. *European Journal Surgery* **161**: 725–7.

42. Fukino O, Tamai H, Fujii S, *et al.* (1983). A study of thyroid function after subtotal thyroidectomy for Graves' disease: particularly on TRH tests, T_3 suppression tests and antithyroid antibodies in euthyroid patients. *Acta Endocrinologica* **103**: 28–33.

43. Werga-Kjellman P, Zedenius J, Tallstedt L, Traisk F, Lundell G, Wallin G (2001). Surgical treatment of hyperthyroidism: a ten year experience. *Thyroid* **11**: 187–92.

44. Perrild H, Jacobsen BB (1996). Thyrotoxicosis in childhood. *European Journal of Endocrinology* **134**: 678–9.

45. AACE Thyroid Task Group (2002). American Association of Clinical Endocrinologists (AACE) medical guidelines for clinical practice for the evaluation and treatment of hyperthyroidism and hypothyroidism. *Endocrine Practice* **8**(6): 458–69.

46. Wesche MF, Tiel-Van Buul MM, Lips P, *et al.* (2001). A randomised trial comparing levothyroxine with radioactive iodine in the treatment of sporadic nontoxic goiter. *Journal of Clinical Endocrinology and Metabolism* **86**: 998–1005.

Appendix 3.1: Suggested algorithm for patients with thyrotoxicosis

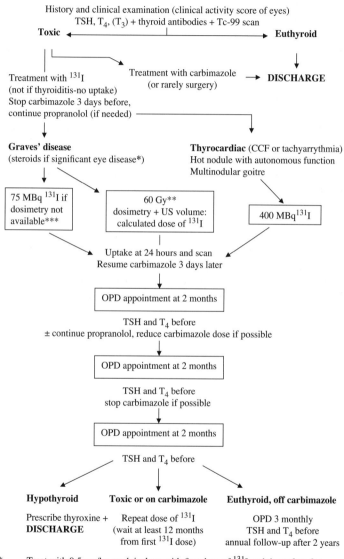

History and clinical examination (clinical activity score of eyes)
TSH, T_4, (T_3) + thyroid antibodies + Tc-99 scan

Toxic ← ⟶ **Euthyroid**

Treatment with ^{131}I
(not if thyroiditis-no uptake)
Stop carbimazole 3 days before,
continue propranolol (if needed)

Treatment with carbimazole
(or rarely surgery) → **DISCHARGE**

Graves' disease
(steroids if significant eye disease*)

Thyrocardiac (CCF or tachyarrythmia)
Hot nodule with autonomous function
Multinodular goitre

75 MBq ^{131}I if
dosimetry not
available***

60 Gy**
dosimetry + US volume:
calculated dose of ^{131}I

400 MBq^{131}I

Uptake at 24 hours and scan
Resume carbimazole 3 days later

OPD appointment at 2 months

TSH and T_4 before
± continue propranolol, reduce carbimazole dose if possible

OPD appointment at 2 months

TSH and T_4 before
stop carbimazole if possible

OPD appointment at 2 months

TSH and T_4 before

Hypothyroid

Prescribe thyroxine +
DISCHARGE

Toxic or on carbimazole

Repeat dose of ^{131}I
(wait at least 12 months
from first ^{131}I dose)

Euthyroid, off carbimazole

OPD 3 monthly
TSH and T_4 before
annual follow-up after 2 years

*　　Treat with 0.5 mg/kg prednisolone with first dose of ^{131}I and thereafter for
　　3 months

**　　Patients with large thyroids detected on ultrasound or prolonged treatment
　　with antithyroids for at least 2 years should receive 120 Gy.

***　　Note that Royal College of Physicians guidelines recommend 400–500 MBq
　　for all patients with Graves' and not just thyrocardiac. See also discussion
　　(section 'Typical doses' above)

Chapter 4

Malignant thyroid disease: use of [131]I

Sue E.M. Clarke, Ujjal Mallick

4.1 Background to use

4.1.1 History

The treatment of differentiated thyroid cancer with ^{131}I radioiodine has a long history. Early reports of the use of radioiodine for therapy appeared in the 1940s[1]. In 1967, Pochin reviewed the use of ^{131}I radioiodine in malignant thyroid disease[2] and identified that 80% of differentiated tumours showed radioiodine uptake. He also observed that papillary and follicular cancers showed similar uptake and response to ^{131}I radioiodine. Beierwaltes, in 1986 reviewed the results of ^{131}I radioiodine therapy in the University of Michigan and noted a threefold survival benefit in patients with metastatic disease treated with ^{131}I radioiodine[3]. A further review by Mazzaferri in 1987 confirmed the therapeutic benefit of radioiodine in patients with tumours greater than 1–1.5 cm in size[4].

The development of guidelines is leading to the standardization of protocols[5–7], although the evidence base for these guidelines remains deficient of large prospective controlled studies.

4.1.2 Pathology

Papillary thyroid cancer is the most common form of differentiated cancer, accounting for approximately 65% of all thyroid carcinomas. They occur more commonly in women. Fine needle aspiration of a papillary thyroid cancer is usually diagnostic as the tumour cells demonstrate typical features of intranuclear grooving and 'orphan Annie' nuclei. Papillary cancers may be found as unexpected asymptomatic lesions in patients undergoing thyroid surgery for benign disease. They are not infrequently multifocal, and spread into cervical lymph nodes is often discovered at the time of presentation. Distant metastases to lung and bone occur less frequently than with follicular tumours. Papillary cancers tend to develop in the third and fourth decades of life. While some pure papillary tumours do not take up iodine, those with follicular elements generally do so and ^{131}I may be used to treat local and distant metastatic spread.

Follicular thyroid cancers are diagnosed when capsular breakthrough of a follicular tumour is demonstrated. They cannot therefore be diagnosed by fine needle aspiration and lobectomy or total thyroidectomy is required in order to make the diagnosis.

Compared with papillary cancers, follicular thyroid cancers tend to occur in an older population, peaking in the fourth and fifth decades of life. Unlike papillary cancers, they metastasize more commonly to bone and lungs. Liver metastases are rare in both follicular and papillary cancers.

While the majority of follicular cancers take up ^{131}I radioiodine at the time of presentation, de-differentiation may occur, and these de-differentiated tumours being more aggressive frequently lose their ability to take up ^{131}I radioiodine. The Hurthle cell variant of follicular cancer is uncommon but is distinguished by the fact that only 10% of these tumours take up ^{131}I radioiodine.

As medullary thyroid cancers and lymphomas do not take up iodine, ^{131}I radioiodine plays no part in their management.

A number of classification systems exist offering prognostic information such as the AMES classification[8] and the MACIS scoring system[9].

4.1.3 ^{131}I Radioiodine

^{131}I has a physical half-life of 8.04 days, which is well suited to the biological half-life of iodine in patients with differentiated thyroid cancer. The median energy beta-particle emission ($E_{max} = 0.61$ mev) with a path length of about 0.5 mm in tissue, ensures an intracellular radiation dose following the cellular internalization of ^{131}I. The gamma emissions of ^{131}I have both benefits and disadvantages. Gamma-ray emissions facilitate gamma-camera imaging, which enables tracer doses of ^{131}I to be used diagnostically and for dosimetry calculations, and also permits post-therapy imaging to confirm uptake of the therapy dose in all known tumour sites.

The high-energy gamma emissions, however, contribute to the unwanted whole-body radiation burden associated with radionuclide therapy and also to the radiation protection problems for the staff and the patients' relatives.

^{131}I Radioiodine, like ordinary iodine, is transported into the thyroid cells and thyroid cancer cells by the sodium iodide symporter protein (NIS). In recent years, NIS has been cloned[10] and *in vitro* and *in vivo* studies have given new insights into iodide transport mechanisms and their defects[11,12]. The iodine pump increases in the presence of iodine deficiency and under thyroid-stimulating hormone (TSH) stimulation. However, the expression of this symporter in thyroid cancer is always decreased and the tumour tissues therefore, take up less iodine compared with normal thyroid cells.

4.2 **Clinical indications**

[131]I Radioiodine plays a key role in the management of most differentiated thyroid cancers. [131]I Radioiodine is routinely used for the ablation of remnant thyroid tissue and is subsequently used, if necessary, to treat recurrent disease. An overview is shown in Fig. 4.1.

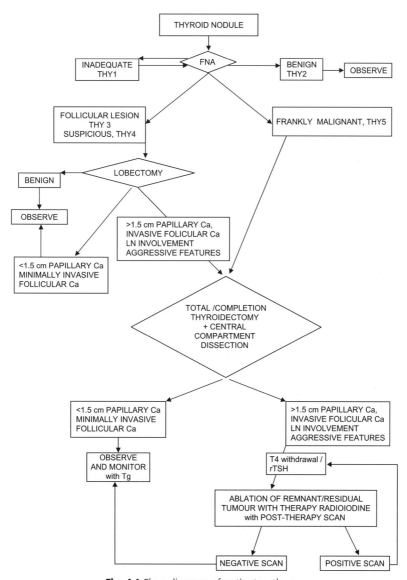

Fig. 4.1 Flow diagram of patient pathway.

4.2.1 Ablation of thyroid remnant

The optimal management for patients having thyroid cancer diagnosed either by fine needle aspiration or at the time of surgery is total thyroidectomy. This may be achieved by a one-stage or a two-stage procedure. Despite careful surgery, however, it is extremely common to demonstrate small residues of normal thyroid tissue on postoperative imaging.

The data demonstrating an outcome advantage to complete ablation of normal thyroid tissue are unclear. While some series have demonstrated a reduction in relapse rate in patients treated with ^{131}I radioiodine postsurgery[13–15], others have failed to show any outcome benefit of radioiodine ablation[16,17]. Sawka *et al.* have conducted a review and meta-analysis of the literature on remnant ablation. They found the data conflicting between studies in low-risk patients, which they attributed to the variations in administered activity and the length of follow-up[18]. Tubiana[19] and Mazaferri and Kloos[20] have clearly demonstrated a benefit in outcome in patients with poorer prognostic features such as tumours over 1.5 cm. Debate continues as to the role of ^{131}I radioiodine in the management of patients with primary tumours less than 1–1.5 cm, particularly those tumours discovered incidentally during surgery for benign goitre.

Ablation of normal thyroid tissue undoubtedly aids follow-up in the following ways:

1. Achieving a negative iodine tracer scan following complete ablation facilitates the interpretation of the subsequent radioiodine tracer scans and the appearance of iodine uptake in the neck subsequent to successful ablation can be reliably interpreted as recurrent tumour.

2. As serum thyroglobulin levels play a key role in the follow-up of patients with differentiated thyroid cancer the achievement of undetectable thyroglobulin levels by total thyroid remnant ablation makes subsequent elevations of thyroglobulin levels interpretable as recurrent disease.

3. As normal thyroid tissue will trap iodine more efficiently than will tumour cells, ^{131}I radioiodine therapy will be less immediately effective if recurrences occur as most of the treatment dose will be taken up by the remnant rather than the tumour recurrence.

4. Lung metastases may not be visible on a tracer iodine scan if there is persisting normal thyroid tissue[21].

4.2.2 Treatment of remnant and recurrent differentiated thyroid cancer

After successful ablation of thyroid tissue with either surgery alone or a combination of surgery and ^{131}I, the subsequent demonstration of focal areas of ^{131}I radioiodine uptake on whole-body imaging is strongly suggestive of metastatic or recurrent thyroid tumour. The normal pattern of radioiodine by distribution, however, must be taken into account when interpreting a whole-body scan. Activity is commonly seen in the salivary glands, nasopharynx, stomach, bowel, and bladder. Care should also be taken to ensure that artefacts are not interpreted as focal areas of recurrent tumour. As ^{131}I radioiodine is secreted in the saliva, contamination of pocket handkerchiefs is a not uncommon problem and may lead to a false-positive interpretation of a whole-body scan if care is not taken to ensure that no contaminated object is imaged (Fig. 4.2). Similarly, urine contamination of underclothes may cause artefacts in the region of the pelvis. [131]I radioiodine will successfully identify sites of both soft tissue and bone recurrence and may be the first indication of lung metastases. Micrometastatic disease in the lung, detected by radioiodine scans only and subsequently treated is associated with good long-term survival. Even with

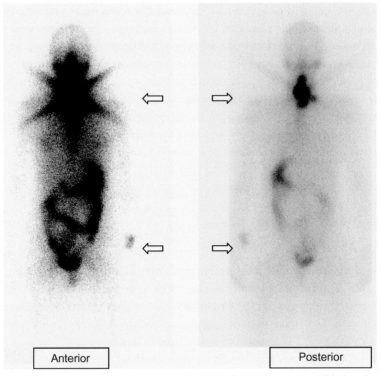

Anterior

Posterior

Fig. 4.2 Whole body post therapy radioiodine scan following 3.7 GBq ablation dose. High uptake in remnant thyroid tissue is noted (arrow) with radioiodine contamination of handkerchief noted (arrow).

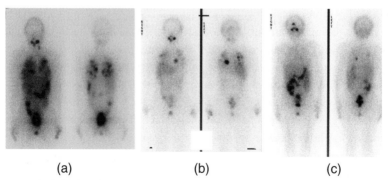

(a)   (b)   (c)

Fig. 4.3 Whole body radioiodine scans: (a) December 1995 showing intense uptake in diffuse lung micrometastases and macrometastases; (b) March 2001 following three treatments with 5.5 GBq radioiodine; (c) November 2001 showing marked improvement in micrometastatic disease but persisting uptake in two foci of macrometastatic disease

macrometastases, although the survival and the response is less, long-term control is still possible (Fig. 4.3).

[131]I radioiodine has also been used as blind treatment in patients with raised thyroglobulin and negative ^{131}I iodine tracer scan. Several theories that have been published showing that blind treatment in a proportion of these patients may be helpful. However, there is variation in approach and it is currently suggested that a selective approach is used rather than giving blind treatment to each and every patient with the risk of long-term radiation damage to the salivary glands and the possibility of second malignancies. The dose for this approach may be limited to 3.7 GBq (100 mCi) to reduce the dose to the lungs from undetected micrometastases.

4.3 **Dose considerations**

4.3.1 **Ablation**

One of the main problems of dosimetry calculations for radioiodine thyroid ablation is the stunning effect of the tracer dose before administration of therapy activity. There is now literature evidence confirming that even relatively low tracer doses of radioiodine will significantly reduce the uptake of a subsequent therapy dose[22,23]. It is therefore recommended that doses of 185 MBq or less are used for the tracer scan to minimize the stunning effect of the tracer dose. In an excellent review, Kalinyak and McDougall have reviewed the evidence for and against stunning. They conclude that some of the conflicting data in the literature may be due to a qualitative rather than a quantitative assessment of radioiodine images in some studies. Stunning appears to be less of a problem if the therapy is given within a week of the tracer scan[24]. New techniques are currently being researched. Park *et al.*[25] are currently exploring the use of high doses of ^{123}I iodine with imaging up to 24 hours postadministration to determine the presence of remnant thyroid and to perform uptake measurements for dosimetry calculations. Further data are required to determine whether the substitution of ^{123}I will improve the efficacy of the subsequent therapy dose and reduce the number of ablation doses required, thereby reducing the requirement for admission with both cost savings and improvement in convenience to the patient. Blake *et al.* have demonstrated that a ^{99m}Tc scan instead of a tracer radioiodine scan will allow the assessment of remnant size prior to radioiodine ablation and improve first time ablation rates[26] (Fig. 4.4).

There is now an increasing practice of undertaking ablation therapy without any pretreatment imaging to avoid the stunning issues.

When considering the ablation dose to be used there are, essentially, two approaches.

Empiric fixed doses

Within this strategic approach there have been two schools, one advocating high fixed administered activities commonly used throughout Europe and the other advocating low fixed activities. Wu *et al.* demonstrated that dividing a 4.4 GBq ablation dose into three fractions at weekly intervals led to an overall mean reduction in uptake of 81% compared with predicted uptake calculated from tracer studies[27]. They suggest that intratherapeutic stunning may be occurring. In the USA, 30 mCi (1000 MBq) is commonly used as this dose

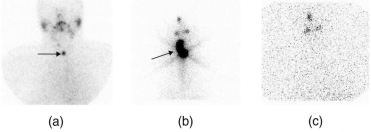

(a)   (b)   (c)

Fig. 4.4 (a) ^{99m}Tc thyroid scan of neck pre-radioiodine ablation showing small remnant of thyroid tissue (arrow); (b) [131]I postablation scan of neck following a 3.7 GBq dose confirming uptake in remnant thyroid (arrow); (c) [131]I tracer scan 6 months after ablation confirming successful ablation of remnant.

may be given as an outpatient. de Groot and Reilly[28] have shown that this leads to ablation in only 60% of cases, while Arad et al.[29] have reported on the use of fractionated doses using 30–50 mCi doses at weekly intervals. The success rate is disappointing, however, with only 25% of patients being ablated. In Europe, larger ablation doses are generally used with 3–3.7 GBq being the standard dose[30].

A few small trials and one meta-analysis have been done. The results are varied. It would appear that if the remnant size is small, a low dose is equally effective as a high dose[31]. Bal et al., in a larger study in India, have prospectively compared the success of using single ablation doses of 25 or 50 mCi (0.9 or 1.8 GBq) of radioiodine in a large series and found no significant difference in ablation success between the two activities[32]. A prospective study is to be undertaken in the UK and France where patients will be randomized to high versus low dosage in a large number of patients in a randomized trial setting.

Quantitative dosimetry

Maxon et al. has suggested that the delivery of 30,000 cGy to the remnant is necessary for adequate ablation and for lymph node metastases 8500 cGy is necessary[33]. Complex dosimetric calculations have been used but most centres are not able to perform these and the estimate of size of the remnant required for such calculations is notoriously prone to error.

Assessment of the completeness of ablation is a subject of debate. One of the accepted methods of assessing ablation is to assess the uptake in the neck in a diagnostic scan at least 6 months after ablation. Values of <0.1% of the administered dose are considered to indicate successful ablation.

4.3.2 Treatment of remnant or recurrent disease

As with remnant ablation, several approaches are available. One is empiric fixed doses of ^{131}I radioiodine, an approach favoured in many centres as being cost-effective and avoiding the requirement for tracer dosimetric studies with the problems of stunning. The range of fixed doses recommended for metastatic disease varies from 5 to 6.2 GBq ^{131}I radioiodine for nodal disease, for pulmonary metastases 6.2–7.4 GBq and for bone metastases 7.4 GBq as recommended by Beierwaltes. Menzel et al. has adopted a more aggressive approach of 11.1 GBq ^{131}I radioiodine at 3-month interval[34].

The advantage of a fixed dose is the ease, convenience and long experience of use. However, it is impossible to say whether an adequate dose is delivered and whether sublethal doses make future doses ineffective. The second approach is the use of a dosimetrically determined dosage. Centres using dosimetric methods to estimate the dose for individual patients base their dose on uptake and retention measurement obtained from the tracer scan or alternatively blood and urine collections and whole-body counting after tracer dose[35]. One approach utilizes so-called BEL dosimetry, which calculates the dose to the blood from a tracer study. Doses are selected to give a maximum of 2 Gy to the blood, with no more than 4.4 GBq retained in the whole body at 48 hours[36,37]. Doses of up to 16.65 MBq (450 mCi) have been used with no permanent suppression of bone marrow observed. Benua and Leeper[38], however, have shown that average values of radiation delivered to the blood are significantly less than the predicted measurements after tracer doses. This observed fact obviously raises the whole question as to the value of estimating doses following dosimetry calculations.

Maxon et al. have advocated lesion based dosimetry rather than whole body or blood dosimetry[39]. Maxon has determined that a good result occurs if a dose of 8.5 Gy to the lymph nodes was achieved but if the dose was less than 3.5 Gy, there was a reduced chance of a successful outcome. It has been proposed by this group that ^{125}I radioiodine may be a more effective radioisotope for therapy for micrometastases[40].

The problems of accurately defining the size of a lesion and the kinetics and distribution of iodine within the lesion have been well reviewed by Van Nostrand et al.[41]

Kosal et al.[42] have shown that doses ranging from 400 to 29,000 rads may be delivered to the tumour using administered doses of 150–170 mCi. O'Connell et al. have used ^{124}I iodine positron emission tomography (PET) in an attempt to more accurately define the volume of recurrent disease and have found that absorbed doses in excess of 100 Gy were found to eradicate cervical node metastases. Metastases that did not respond were calculated to have received less than 20 Gy[43]. More recently, Eschmann et al. have further explored the possibilities of using PET to facilitate lesion dosimetry[44]. Sgouros et al. have developed three-dimensional imaging based dosimetry, which is patient specific using ^{124}I iodine PET. They have used post-therapy imaging to demonstrate that mean absorbed dose values for individual tumours range from 1.2 to 540 Gy with absorbed doses within tumours ranging from 0.3 to 4000 Gy[45].

Flux et al. have looked at the implications of random error in dosimetric calculations[46] and Luster et al. have identified changes in iodine kinetics between tracer studies performed under recombinant human TSH (rhTSH) stimulation and therapy doses performed with thyroxine withdrawal[47].

The importance of an agreed approach to dosimetric calculations is now recognized, which must take account of current technology without increasing inappropriately the interval before treatment is undertaken, considering the possible effects of stunning and minimizing the inconvenience to the patient of multiple hospital visits.

The absence of randomized trials and the complexity of the measurements required to calculate doses has led to the adoption of empiric doses for treatment of metastatic thyroid cancer in routine practice.

4.4 **Patient preparation and precautions**

Before undertaking an ^{131}I radioiodine tracer scan, the patient should be asked to discontinue thyroid replacement hormone. If the patient is taking thyroxine, a minimum of 4 weeks off treatment is required to ensure adequate TSH levels at the time of imaging. If the patient is taking triiodothyronine, then a 2-week cessation of therapy is adequate. TSH levels must be measured at the time of undertaking ^{131}I imaging to ensure the patient's compliance with instructions and to confirm an adequate rise in TSH before a scan is interpreted as negative.

rhTSH administration has been shown to be virtually as effective as thyroid hormone withdrawal in preparing patients for repeat tracer radioiodine imaging with significant improvement in patient quality of life in two large multicentre studies[48,49]. rhTSH is now licensed in Europe and the USA as an alternative to thyroxine withdrawal for preparing patients for tracer imaging. The rhTSH is given as two intramuscular injections on sequential days. The tracer radioiodine dose is given on day 3 and the scan performed, together with a thyroglobulin measurement on day 5.

Many studies have now been reported confirming the successful use of rhTSH prior to ablation therapy and radioiodine therapy of recurrent disease[50]. It has been shown, however, that the effective half-life of radioiodine is shorter with rhTSH preparation compared with thyroxine withdrawal. It is postulated that higher therapy doses may therefore be required[51]. rhTSH is now licensed for therapeutic use in the ablation of thyroid remnant but not, as yet, for the treatment of remnant or recurrent disease. Its use in treatment on a named patient basis is now becoming acceptable following the publication of recent work from New York, which has suggested the use of recombinant TSH in patients who have a poor TSH response or in those in whom the time delay necessitated in stopping thyroid hormone replacement is clinically unacceptable[52]. Patients with aggressive disease in whom prolonged TSH stimulation may stimulate tumour growth should also be considered for rhTSH rather than thyroxine withdrawal.

The use of low iodine diet in the period before tracer imaging will further enhance the avidity of thyroid tumour recurrence for ^{131}I radioiodine.

The amount of ^{131}I radioiodine to be administered for the tracer scan again varies. The justification for a low tracer dose regimen is the avoidance of possible stunning effects of the tracer dose on a subsequent therapy dose. There is little evidence in the literature, however, to suggest that the stunning effects seen in the normal thyroid also occurs in thyroid tumour cells and as tumour cells are known to be less radio-sensitive than normal cells, it may be postulated that the stunning effect is less important when considering treatment of recurrence compared with ablation of thyroid remnants. The advantage of a high tracer dose (up to 400 MBq) is the higher sensitivity for detecting recurrent disease. The increase in sensitivity with dose is clearly evidenced by the fact that post-therapy scans not uncommonly show lesions that were not detected on a tracer scan[53]. Siddiqi *et al.* have compared the sensitivity of a whole body ^{131}I radioiodine tracer scan with a ^{123}I radioiodine scan in a small series and showed good concordance between the two methods[54].

Schlumberger[55] recommended a protocol which takes into account the lower sensitivity of the low-dose tracer scan regimen. He proposes that patients with an elevated thyroglobulin level and a normal tracer scan should receive a therapy dose of ^{131}I radioiodine. Experience indicated that 50% of patients thus treated show uptake on the post-therapy scan (Fig. 4.5).

A patient in whom a tracer scan is performed will be required to observe precautions as for a ^{131}I radioiodine dose for thyrotoxicosis if they are scanned as an outpatient. Again, extreme care must be taken to ensure that if the patient is a female, they are neither pregnant nor breast-feeding, as both conditions remain absolute contraindications to tracer scanning and subsequent therapy.

In those patients in whom the tracer scan confirms a focal area or areas of recurrence, therapy doses of ^{131}I may be administered. For this, the patient must be admitted into a designated room with en-suite bathroom facilities. Daily monitoring of the patient is required to ensure that the patient is not discharged until the radiation levels fall to those acceptable under national regulations[56]. Visitors must be kept to a minimum, with visiting times being restricted to not more than 10 minutes per day.

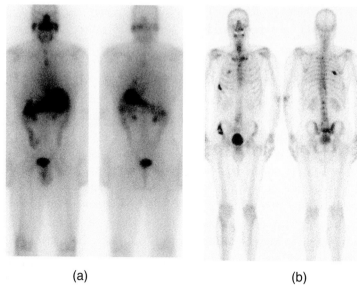

(a)   (b)

Fig. 4.5 Post-therapy radioiodine scan (a) after blind 5.5 GBq dose radioiodine in patient with rapidly rising thyroglobulin levels showing no therapeutic uptake (oesophageal activity noted). Bone scan (b) shows widespread non-radioiodine avid bone metastases. Patient's disease progressed rapidly and patient died within 1 year.

4.5 Side-effects following ^{131}I radioiodine therapy

4.5.1 Acute

As ^{131}I radioiodine is taken up and secreted by the salivary glands as well as by recurrent thyroid tumour sites, a significant radiation dose is received by the salivary glands. Becciolini *et al.*[57] have calculated the absorbed dose to the salivary glands based on external beam data to range between 0.24 and 2.29 Gy. Patients are commonly aware of swelling and mild discomfort in the region of the salivary gland in the immediate post-therapy period and complain of alteration in taste with a metallic taste frequently noted. While these symptoms generally resolve after the first one or two treatments, subsequent treatments may result in a permanent reduction in salivary flow and a consequent dryness of the mouth and impaired sensation of taste[58]. Attempts to reduce the radiation dose to the salivary glands have been made by suggesting patients chew gum or suck citrus sweets for 24 hours following therapy in order to increase salivary flow and thereby increase the rate of excretion of ^{131}I radioiodine from the salivary gland area. There are few data, however, to confirm the efficacy of this recommendation and Nakada *et al.* have demonstrated that increasing salivary flow using citrus sweets in the first 24 hours after treatment increases salivary gland damage[59].

Radiation doses to the bladder are minimized by ensuring a high urine output during the admission for therapy.

Some patients complain of nausea in the first 48 hours after therapy. This appears to be idiosyncratic. It is readily treated with conventional anti-emetics.

Transient episodes of marrow suppression have been observed in patients with widespread bone metastases. This appears to be a greater problem in patients of West African and West Indian background.

Transient impairment of testicular function has been demonstrated by Pacini *et al.* They concluded that approximately 25% of patients treated with ^{131}I suffered no alterations in follicle-stimulating hormone levels, whereas the remainder had transient rises in hormone levels. Patients treated repeatedly over a prolonged period had a reduced sperm count. Consideration should therefore be given to sperm banking in young men with metastatic thyroid cancer who are likely to require multiple treatments with radioiodine.

4.5.2 Long term

Long-term side-effects of ^{131}I therapy, apart from sialadenitis and xerostomia, are remarkably few. In patients with widespread lung metastases, particularly those with miliary metastases, caution must be taken in determining the dose to be administered in view of the risk of radiation fibrosis[61].

Leukaemia has been reported as a complication in patients receiving aggressive therapy with total administered doses exceeding 1 Ci with intervals of less than 6 months between treatments[61].

Cancer of the bladder is a theoretical long-term complication of ^{131}I radioiodine therapy given the radiation doses to the bladder in the early phases of treatment. Few reports of cases of cancer of the bladder have been made, although Edmonds and Smith describe cases in patients who have received a cumulative dose of over 1 Ci[61]. Hall *et al.*[62], using the Swedish Cancer Registry, have followed a large cohort of patients with cancer of the thyroid treated with ^{131}I radioiodine, but have failed to show any long-term increase in incidence of solid tumours (including bladder tumours). Rubino *et al.*, however, in a recent paper have reported on the appearance of secondary primary malignancies in thyroid cancer patients[63].

4.6 Adjunctive treatment

Patients who are found to have extensive tumour spread to soft tissues outside the thyroid gland at the time of primary surgery may be considered for external beam radiotherapy following surgery as an adjunct to ^{131}I radioiodine therapy. It is optimal to undertake ^{131}I radioiodine treatment before external beam therapy to avoid radiation damage to thyroid remnant and residual thyroid tumour cells, which may reduce the efficacy of the ^{131}I radioiodine dose. Local radiotherapy to sites of painful bone metastases should also be considered for bone pain palliation.

Chemotherapy has been shown to be generally ineffective in treating patients with recurrent disease.

4.7 Innovative ways of using ^{131}I

At the Institut Gustave Roussy in France ^{131}I has been used to aid detection of disease intraoperatively by using a gamma probe after administration of ^{131}I[64].

Several agents have been used to increase the effectiveness of radioiodine therapy. Lithium had been used to reduce the outflow of iodine from thyroid cells. Retinoic acid had been used to redifferentiate refractory thyroid cancer cells and increase their iodine uptake. However, the benefit of this is doubtful. Histone deacetylase inhibitors have also been used to augment radioiodine accumulation in non-iodine avid thyroid cancer cells[65].

A flow diagram indicates the patient pathway following the diagnosis of thyroid cancer (Fig. 4.5).

References

1. Williams RH, Tovery BT, Jaffe H (1949). Radiotherapies. *American Journal of Medicine* **7**: 702–4.

2. Pochin EE (1967). Prospects from the treatment of thyroid carcinoma with radioiodine. *Clinical Radiology* **18**: 113–35.

3. Beierwaltes WH (1986). Carcinoma of the thyroid—radionuclide diagnosis, therapy and follow up. *Clinics in Oncology* **5**: 23–37.

4. Mazzaferri EL (1987). Papillary thyroid carcinoma: factors influencing prognosis and current therapy. *Seminars in Oncology* **14**: 315–32.

5. Mazzaferri E (1999). NCCN Thyroid Carcinoma Practice Guidelines. *Oncology* **13**: 391–442.

6. Meier DA, Brill DA, Becker DV, Clarke SE, Silberstein EB, Royal HD, Balan HR (2002). Procedure Guidelines for the therapy of thyroid disease with radioiodine. *Journal of Nuclear Medicine* **43**: 856–61.

7. Guidelines for the Management of Thyroid Cancer in Adults, British Thyroid Association and Royal College of Physicians (2002). www.british-thyroid-association.org.

8. Cady B, Rossi R (1988). A expanded view of risk group definition in differentiated thyroid carcinoma. *Surgery* **104**: 947–953.

9. Hay ID, Bergstrahl EJ, Goellner JR, *et al.* (1993). Predicting Outcome in Papillary thyroid carcinoma: development of reliable prognostic scoring system in a cohort of 1779 patients surgically treated in one institution during 1940–1989. *Surgery* **114**: 1050–8.

10. Dai G, Levy O, Carrasco N (1996). Cloning and characterization of the thyroid iodide transporter. *Nature* **379**: 458–60.

11. Filetti S, Bidart J-M, Arturi F, Caillou B, Russo D, Schlumberger M (1999). Sodium/iodide symporter: a key transport system in thyroid cancer cell metabolism. *European Journal of Endocrinology* **141**: 443–57.

12. Dadachova E, Carrasco N (2004). The Na+/I symporter: Imaging and therepaeutic applications. *Seminars in Nuclear Medicine* **34**: 23–31.

13. Beierwaltes WH (1987). Carcinoma of the thyroid. Radionuclide diagnosis, therapy and follow-up. *Clinical Oncology* **5**: 23–7.

14. Mazzaferri EL (1987). Papillary thyroid carcinoma: factors influencing prognosis and current therapy. *Seminars in Oncology* **14**: 315–32.

15. Mazzaferri EL, Kloos RD (2001). Current approaches to primary therapy for papillary and follicular thyroid cancer. *Journal of Clinical Endocrinology and Metabolism* **86**: 1447–63.

16. Tubiana M (1985). Long term results and prognostic factors with differentiated thyroid carcinoma. *Cancer* **55**: 794–804.

17. McConahey WM (1986). Papillary thyroid cancer treated at the Mayo Clinic, 1946 through 1970: initial manifestations, pathologic findings, therapy and outcome. *Mayo Clinical Proceedings* **61**: 978–96.

18. Sawka AM, Thephamongkhol K, Brouwers M, Thabane L, Browman G, Gerstein H, (2004). A systematic review and meta-analysis of the effectiveness of radioiodine remant ablation for well differentiated thyroid cancer. *Journal of Clinical Endocrinology and Metabolism* **89**: 3662–4.

19. Tubiana M (1982). Thyroid cancer. In Beckers C (ed.) *Thyroid diseases*, pp. 182–227. Paris: Pergamon Press.

20. Mazzaferri EL, Kloos R (2001). Clinical Review 128: Current approaches to primary therapy for papillary and follicular thyroid cancer. *Journal of Clinical Endocrinology and Metabolism* **86**: 1447–63.

21. Bal CS, Kumar A, Chandra P, Dwivedi SN, Mukhopadhyaya S (2004). Is chest X-ray or high resolution CT of the chest sufficient investigation to detect pulmonary metastases in paediatric differentiated thyroid cancer. *Thyroid* **14**: 217–25.

22. Jeevanram RK, Shah DH, Sharma SM, Ganatra RD (1986). Influence of initial large dose on subsequent uptake of therapeutic radioiodine in thyroid cancer patients. *Nuclear Medicine and Biology* **13**: 277–9.

23. Park JM (1992). Stunned thyroid after high dose 131-I imaging. *Clinical Nuclear Medicine* **17**: 501–2.

24. Kalinyak JE, Mcdougall IR (2004). Whole body scanning with radionuclides of iodine, and the controversy of 'thyroid stunning'. *Nuclear Medicine Communications* **25**: 883–9.

25. Park HM, Perkins OW, Edmonson JW, Schnute RB, Manatunga A (1994). Influence of diagnostic radioiodines on the uptake of ablative doses of iodine131. *Thyroid* **4**: 49–54.

26. Blake GM, Patel R, Prescod N, Clarke SEM (1998). Thyroid stunning by a 131I tracer scan prior to radioiodine ablation for thyroid cancer. *Nuclear Medicine Communications* **19**: 158.

27. Wu H, Hseu H, Lin W, Wang S, Liu Y (2005). Decreased uptake after fractionated ablative doses of iodine-131. *Eur J Nucl Med Mol Imaging* **32**: 167–73.

28. de Groot LJ, Reilly M (1982). Comparison of 30 and 50 mCi doses for 131-Iodine ablation. *Annals Internal Medicine* **96**: 51–2.

29. Arad E, Flannery K, Wilson G, O'Mara R (1990). Fractionated doses of radioiodine ablation of post surgical thyroid tissue remnants. *Clinical Nuclear Medicine* **16**: 676–7.

30. Kuni CC, Klingensmith WC (1980). Failure of low doses of ^{131}I to ablate residual thyroid tissue following surgery for thyroid cancer. *Radiology* **137**: 773–4.

31. Mallick Ujjal K, Charalambous H (2004). Current issues in the management of differentiated thyroid cancer. *Nuclear Medicine Communications* **25**: 873–81.

32. Bal CS, Kumar A, Pant GS (2004). Radioiodine dose for remnant ablation in differentiated thyroid carcinoma: a randomized clinical trial in 500 patients. *Journal of Clinical Endocrinology and Metabolism* **89**: 1666–73.

33. Maxon HR, Englaro EE, Thomas SR, Hertzberg VS, Hinnefeld JD, Chen LS, Smith H, Cummings D, Aden MD (1992). Radioiodine-131 Therapy for well-differentiated thyroid cancer—a quantitative radiation dosimetric approach: outcome and validation in 85 patients. *Journal of Nuclear Medicine* **33**: 1132–6.

34. Menzel C, Grunwald A, Schomburg A, Palmedo H, Bender H, Spath G, Biersack H (1996). 'High dose' radioiodine therapy in advanced differentiated thyroid carcinoma. *Journal of Nuclear Medicine* **37**: 1496–503.

35. Maxon HR, Thomas SR, Hertzberg VS (1983). Relation between effective radiation dose and outcome of radioiodine therapy for thyroid cancer. *New England Journal of Medicine* **309**: 937–41.

36. Benua RS, Cieale NR, Sonenberg M (1962). The relation of radioiodine dose to results and complications in the treatment of metastatic thyroid cancer. *American Journal of Roentgenology, Radiation Therapy and Nuclear Medicine* **87**: 171–82.

37. Leeper RD, Shimaoka K (1980). Treatment of metastatic thyroid cancer. *Clinical Endocrinology and Metabolism* **9**: 383–404.

38. Benua RS, Leeper RD (1986). A method and rationale for treating metastatic thyroid carcinoma with the largest safe dose of I-131. In: Medeiros-Neto G, Gaitan E (eds). *Frontiers in thyroidology*, Vol. 2, pp. 1317–21. New York: Plenum Medical Book Co.

39. Maxon HR, Thomas SR, Samaratunga RC (1997). Dosimetric considerations in the radioiodine treatment of macrometastases and micrometastases from differentiated thyroid cancer. *Thyroid* **7**(2): 183–7.

40. Maxon HR (1999). Quantitative radioiodine therapy in the treatment of differentiated thyroid cancer. *Quarterly Journal of Nuclear Medicine* **43**: 313–23.

41. Van Nostrand D, Atkins F, Yeganeh F, Acio E, Bursaw R, Wartofsky L (2002). Review: dosimetrically determined doses of radioiodine for the treatment of metastatic thyroid carcinoma. *Thyroid* **12**(2): 121–34.

42. Kosal KF, Adler SF, Carey J, Beierwaltes W (1986). Iodine 131 treatment of thyroid cancer: absorbed dose calculated from post therapy scans. *Journal of Nuclear Medicine* **27**: 1207–11.

43. O'Connell ME, Flower MA, Hinton PJ, Harmer CL, McCready VR (1993). Radiation dose assessment in radioiodine therapy. Dose–response relationships in differentiated thyroid cancer using quantitative scanning and PET. *Radiotherapy and Oncology* **28**: 16–26.

44. Eschmann SM, Reischi G, Bilger K, *et al.* (2202). Evaluation of dosimetry of radioiodine therapy in benign and malignant thyroid disorders by means of iodine-124 and PET. *European Journal of Nuclear Medicine and Molecular Imaging* **29**: 760–7.

45. Sgouros G, Kolbert MS, Sheikh A, Pentlow KS, Mun EF, Barth A, Robbins RJ, Larson SM, (2004). Patient specific dosimetry for 131I thyroid cancer therapy using 124 I PET and 3 dimensional internal dosimetry software. *Journal of Nuclear Medicine* **45**: 1366–72.

46. Flux GD, Guy MJ, Beddows R, Pryor M, Flower MA (2002). Estimation and implications of random error in whole-body dosimetry for targeted radionuclide therapy. *Physics in Medicine and Biology* **47**(17): 3211–23.

47. Luster M, Sherman SL, Skarulis MC, *et al.*(2003). Comparison of radioiodine biokinetics following the administration of recombinant human thyroid stimulating hormone and after thyroid hormone withdrawal in the thyroid carcinoma. *Journal of Nuclear Medicine and Molecular Imaging* **44**: 1371–7.

48. Haugen BR, Pacini F, Reiners C (1999). A comparison of recombinant human thyrogen and thyroid hormone withdrawal for the detection of thyroid remnant or cancer. *Journal of Clinical Endocrinology and Metabolism* **84**: 3877–85.

49. Ladenson PW, Braverman LE, Mazzaferri EL (1997). Comparison of administration of recombinant human thyrogen with withdrawal of thyroid hormone for radioactive iodine scanning in patients with thyroid carcinoma. *New England Journal of Medicine* **337**: 888–96.

50. Robbins R (2003). Recombinant human TSH and thyroid cancer management— clinical review. *Journal of Clinical Endocrinology and Metabolism* **88**: 1933–8.

51. Menzel C, Kranert WT, Dobert N, Diehl M, (2003). RhTSH stimulation before radioiodine therapy in thyroid cancer reduces the effective half life of radioiodine. *Journal of Nuclear Medicine* **44**: 1065–8.

52. Braverman LE, Pratt BM, Ebner S, Longcope C (1992). Recombinant human thyrotropin stimulates thyroid function and radioactive iodine uptake in Rhesus monkeys. *Journal of Clinical Endocrinology and Metabolism* **74**: 1135–9.

53. Maxon HR, Thomas SR, Hertzberg VS (1983). Relation between effective radiation dose and outcome of radioiodine therapy for thyroid cancer. *New England Journal of Medicine* **309**: 937–41.

54. Siddiqi A, Foley RR, Britton KE, Sibtain A, Plowman PN, Grossman AB, Monson JP, Besser GM (2001). The role of 123 I diagnostic imaging in the follow up of patients with differentiated thyroid cancer as compared to 131 I scanning: avoidance of negative therapeutic uptake due to stunning. *Clinical Endocrinology* **55**: 515–21.

55. Schlumberger M (1988). Detection and treatment of lung metastases of differentiated thyroid cancer in patients with normal chest X-rays. *Journal of Nuclear Medicine* **29**: 1790–4.

56. Fruhling J (1994). Role of radioactive iodine in the treatment of differentiated thyroid cancer: physiopathological basis, results, considerations from the viewpoint of radioprotection. *Bulletin et Memoires de l'Academie Royale de Medecine de Belgique* **149**: 192–206.

57. Becciolini A, Porciani S, Lanini A, Benucci A, Castagnoli A, Pupi A (1994). Serum amylase and tissue polypeptide antigen as biochemical indicators of salivary gland injury during iodine-131 therapy. *European Journal of Nuclear Medicine* **21**: 1121–5.

58. Kabra R, Prescod N, Allen S, Clarke SEM (2004). Salivary gland function in patients with Ca thyroid treated with radioiodine. *Nuclear Medicine Communications* **25**: 402–3.

59. Nakada K, Ishibashi T, Takei T, *et al.* (2005). Does lemon candy decrease salivary gland damage after radioiodine therapy for thyroid cancer. *Journal of Nuclear Medicine* **46**: 261–6.

60. Pacini F, Gasperi M, Fugazzola L, Cecearelli C, Lippi F, Centoni R, Martino E, Pinehera A (1994). Testicular function in patients with differentiated thyroid carcinoma treated with radioiodine. *Journal of Nuclear Medicine* **35**: 1418–22.

61. Edmonds C, Smith T (1986). The long term hazards of treatment of thyroid cancer with radioiodine. *British Journal of Radiology* **59**: 45–51.

62. Hall P, Holm LE, Lundell GE (1992). Cancer risks in thyroid cancer patients. *British Journal of Cancer* **64**: 159–63.

63. Rubino C, de Vathaire F, Dottorini ME, Hall P, Schvartz C, Couette JE, Dondon MG, Abbas MT, Langlois C, Schlumberger (2003). Second primary malignancies in thyroid cancer patients. *British Journal of Cancer* **89**: 1638–44.

64. Travagli J, Cailleux A, Ricard M *et al.* (1998). Combination of radioiodine (^{131}I) and probe guided surgery for persistent or recurrent thyroid carcinoma. *Journal of Clinical Endocrinology and Metabolism* **83**: 2675–80.

65. Robins RJ, Schlumberger MJ (2005). The evolving role of ^{131}I for the treatment of differentiated thyroid carcinoma. *Journal of Nuclear Medicine* **46**: 1(Suppl.) 28S–37S.

Chapter 5

Neuroendocrine tumours

Jamshed Bomanji, G. Gnanasegaran

5.1 Introduction

Neuroendocrine tumours (NETs) are rare, slow-growing malignancies, which have distinct biological and clinical characteristics. They are derived from neoplastic proliferation of cells of the diffuse neuroendocrine system[1].

NETs account for 0.5% of all malignant tumours and the estimated incidence is approximately 2/100 000 of the population with a predilection for females under the age of 50 years[2]. The most common site is the gastrointestinal tract[2,3]. NETs are well known for producing various hormonal syndromes and for their indolent clinical course in most patients. The therapeutic strategy in neuroendocrine tumours is complex, both due to tumour heterogeneity and to the fact that, although generally slow growing, a significant proportion of these tumours may demonstrate an aggressive nature in their progression[4].

Historically during the 1970s and 1980s chemotherapy was considered the standard treatment of neuroendocrine tumours. During the 1980s both interferon (IFN)-α and somatostatin (SMS) analogue therapies were developed and since then there has been a significant improvement in the management of malignant neuroendocrine tumours[4,5]. Tumours that are localized or have spread regionally to lymph nodes are best managed by surgical resection; however, most NETs are metastatic at first diagnosis. Non-functioning indolent tumours that progress slowly may require no specific intervention until they produce symptoms due to mass effect. Chemotherapy can be offered to these patients but produces a partial remission in about 40% of patients with a median survival of 2 years. Patients positive on octreotide scanning would be suitable for therapy with octreotide-labelled radionuclides[5].

5.2 General principles of radionuclide therapy

Radionuclide therapy is based on the deposition of ionizing radiation in tumours or organ tissues. One of the interesting concepts in radiation oncology is the delivery of high radiation dose to the tumour, while sparing the surrounding and normal tissues. Targeted radionuclide therapy owing to the length of the

Table 5.1 Physical properties of radionuclides used in the treatment of neuroendocrine tumours

---

131Iodine: ^{131}I is a β-emitting radionuclide with (($t_{0.5}$ = 8.04 days), a principal γ-ray of 364 keV (81% abundance) and β particles with a maximum energy of 0.61 MeV and an average energy of 0.192

111Indium: ^{111}In ($t_{0.5}$ = 67 h) imaging is performed over several days. ^{111}In nuclide decays by electron capture with emission of γ photons of 173 and 247 keV (89% and 95% abundance, respectively), which is used in γ scintigraphy

90Yttrium: ^{90}Y is obtained in high-specific activity from ^{90}Sr. ^{90}Y ($t_{0.5}$ = 64 hours) is a β$^-$ emitter, which is the most frequently used radionuclide for targeted radionuclide therapy

177Lutetium: The most frequently used radionuclide of lutetium is ^{177}Lu ($t_{0.5}$ = 160.8 h). It is a short-range β and a γ emitter and the physical characteristics similar to ^{131}I (113 and 208 keV gamma photons). It has an average energy of 148 keV and a maximum range of 1.5 mm

---

emitters, causes a bystander effect by cross firing, thus cells close to the tumour are also killed[6–8]. A radiopharmaceutical, which delivers high radiation to target tissues with minimal collateral damage, would be ideal. Recently, there has been significant effort in development of radiopharmaceuticals to improve tumour targeting together with simultaneous reduction of physiological organ uptake. The choice of radiopharmaceutical depends on the tumour type, characteristics of the radioisotope (Table 5.1), chemical nature of the compound, and biological behaviour of the labelled radiopharmaceutical[7]. Factors, which further influence uptake, include change in blood supply, interstitial pressure, permeability, and increase in the extravascular space[8]. Radionuclide treatment of NETs is mostly carried out with radiolabelled meta-iodobenzylguanidine (mIBG) and SMS analogues[8].

5.3 Neuroendocrine tumours and radionuclide therapy

NETs possess either neuroamine uptake mechanisms or specific receptors at the cell membrane[9], some tumour cells may possess both mechanisms. Radiolabelled-mIBG is transported across the cell membrane dominantly via the neuronal uptake mechanism, while SMS analogues target the specific receptors expressed by these tumours. When a β-emitting radioisotope is coupled to mIBG or a SMS analogue (Table 5.2), it may specifically target tumour cells delivering an effective radiation dose to the target tissue or tumour. The high sensitivity, specificity, and avid uptake of ^{111}In-labelled pentetreotide and ^{123}I-labelled mIBG by the NETs in diagnostic scanning, led

Table 5.2 Radiopharmaceuticals used for radionuclide therapy of neuroendocrine tumours

^{131}I-mIBG (meta-iodobenzylguanidine)
[^{111}In-DTPA^0] –octreotide /^{111}In-pentetreotide
[^{90}Y-DOTA^0, Tyr^3] octreotide (^{90}Y-Dotato, ^{90}Y-SMT-487, Octreother)
[^{90}Y-DOTA]-lanreotide
[^{177}Lu-DOTA^0-Tyr^3-Thr^8] octreotide (^{177}Lu-Dotatate)
[^{90}Y-DOTA]-octreotate

to the development of receptor-targeted therapy. However, it is important to remember that neither of these radiotracers on their own, or in combination, map the full extent of disease[10]. Therefore, some tumour cells will always escape detection and the effects of targeted radionuclide therapy.

5.4 ^{131}I-Meta-iodobenzylguanidine (^{131}I-mIBG) therapy

mIBG is a *meta* isomer of the guanethidine derivative iodobenzylguanidine. Radiolabelled mIBG is commonly used in the diagnosis and treatment of tumours of neural crest origin (Table 5.3). The sensitivity and specificity of radiolabelled mIBG in detecting phaeochromocytoms is >90%, but the detection rate is slightly lower in carcinoid tumours[11,12]. ^{131}I-mIBG therapy is used in patients with phaeochromocytoma, paragangliomas, neuroblastomas, and carcinoids.

As part of the patient selection process (Table 5.4) prior to therapy, a diagnostic scan should be performed to document uptake and retention of

Table 5.3 Indications of targeted radionuclide therapy

^{131}I-mIBG therapy ($^{123/131}$I-mIBG positive tumours)	Radiolabelled somatostatin analogue therapy ^{111}In-pentetreotide positive tumours
Inoperable malignant phaeochromocytoma Inoperable or malignant paraganglioma	Inoperable sympathoadrenal system tumours (phaeochromocytoma, and paraganglioma)
Inoperable or malignant carcinoid tumour	Inoperable functioning gastroenteropancreatic tumours (carcinoid, gastrinoma, insulinoma, glucagonoma, VIPoma, etc.)
Inoperable, malignant medullary thyroid cancer	Inoperable medullary thyroid carcinoma Neuroendocrine tumours of unknown origin

Table 5.4 ^{131}I-mIBG therapy procedure* (Kindly note all the above mentioned protocols are arbitrary and currently there are no strict guidelines)

Eligibility criteria and checklist prior to therapy

1. Patients should have a biopsy proven, inoperable neuroendocrine tumour

2. mIBG positive tumours, documented by quantitative tracer scan

3. Oral potassium iodate or potassium iodide commencing 1 day prior to mIBG therapy and continued for up to 3 days post-therapy

4. Drugs interfering with the uptake and/or retention of [131I]-mIBG should be withdrawn for 1–2 weeks prior to treatment (patients should be stabilized on alternative medication prior to therapy).

5. Patients should receive adequate (written and verbal) information about the procedure and explain the procedure to the patient

6. Written consent must be obtained from the patient

7. Patients and careers should receive specific instruction/information in radiation safety precautions

Procedure

Usual administered activities range between 3.7 and 11.2 GBq (100–300 mCi)

Activity reduction should be considered in patients with myelosuppression and impaired renal function

131I-mIBG, diluted in 50–100 ml saline or glucose solution, in compliance with the manufacturer's instructions, is administered by slow intravenous infusion (45 minutes–4 hours) via an indwelling cannula or central venous line using a lead-shielded infusion system. The infusion line should be flushed at the same rate at the end of the procedure

Vita signs monitoring is essential as mIBG administration may result in unstable blood pressure (BP)

Continuous BP monitoring through out infusion is recommended

Prophylactic antiemetics are advised (ondansetron is the antiemetic of choice)

Reducing or temporarily stopping the 131I-mIBG infusion usually manages unstable hypertension

Patient instruction and precautions

Urinary 131I-mIBG excretion is of particular concern during the first 5 days postadministration

Patients should be advised to observe rigorous hygiene in order to avoid contaminating

Patients should be warned to avoid soiling underclothing

Double toilet flush and hand wash is recommended after urination

Incontinent patients should be catheterized prior to 131I-mIBG administration

Return the waste to the hot lab in nuclear medicine for disposal

Set up radiation protection procedures and appropriate signage on the door

Check the room for contamination after sending the patient home

Table 5.4 131I-mIBG therapy procedure* (Kindly note all the above mentioned protocols are arbitrary and currently there are no strict guidelines) (continued)

Decontaminate the room and make it available for next patient
Post therapy imaging on day 5 post-treatment
Follow-up
Weekly blood count for at least 6 weeks post-therapy
Treatment may be repeated at not less than 6-weekly (adults) intervals, dictated by platelet recovery
Tumour response assessment using conventional radiological or radionuclide methods

123I-mIBG in tumour sites[13,14](Fig. 5.1). Patients with myelosuppression and renal failure are poor candidates for therapy[15]. Care should be taken to avoid drugs interfering with mIBG uptake[16]. Prior to 131I-mIBG therapy thyroid blockade with oral potassium iodide (KI) and perchlorate is necessary to protect the thyroid[15,17,18].

There are no consensual published guidelines for 131I-mIBG dose or dose schedules for palliative therapy. Most literature reports recommend 131I-mIBG doses between 100 and 300 mCi (3.7–11.1GBq) for these tumours[19–22]. Several doses may be required to obtain an objective response and the treatment should not be repeated less than 4–6 weeks.

131I-mIBG therapy is given on an in-patient basis in a dedicated lead-lined room. The infusion is given over a period of 30–60 min in a shielded infusion system[15]. Vital signs are monitored during and 4 hours post-infusion. Post-therapy whole body scans are obtained to document the extent of 131I-mIBG uptake in tumour sites (Fig. 5.2).

Side-effects of 131I-mIBG therapy are minimal (Table 5.5). Nausea and vomiting may occur during the first two days post-therapy, transient myelo-suppression may occur 4–6 weeks post-therapy. Bone marrow suppression is more likely in patients who have bone marrow involvement at the time of 131I-mIBG therapy[14,15,18,19,23,24].

5.4.1 Clinical efficacy of 131I-mIBG therapy

Malignant phaeochromocytoma

In patients with metastatic phaeochromocytoma treatment options are relatively few. Loh *et al.*[13] in their extensive review of the literature in 116 patients with malignant phaeochromocytoma reported an initial sympto-matic improvement in 76% of patients, tumour responses in 30%, and

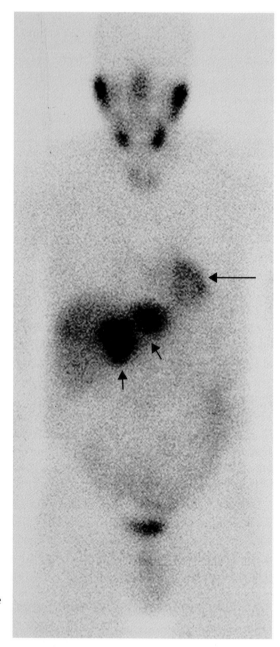

Fig. 5.1 ^{123}I-mIBG scan (anterior view) shows liver metastases (small arrows) in a patient with metastatic carcinoid tumour. Large arrow shows normal cardiac activity.

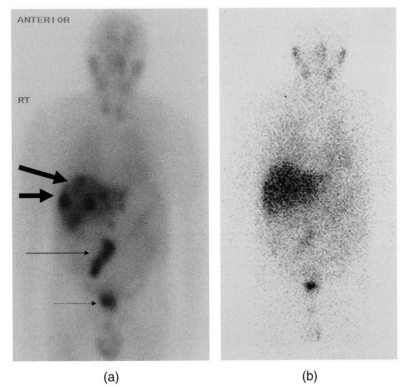

(a)   (b)

Fig. 5.2 (A) 131I-mIBG whole body scan (posterior view) in a patient with metastatic carcinoid tumour treated with 11.1 GBq (300 mCi) of 131I-mIBG. The scan shows good accumulation of activity in liver metastases (large arrows), and a mesenteric mass (small arrows). Excreted activity is seen in bladder (dashed arrow). Patient received a cumulative dose of 33.3 GBq (900 mCi) of 131I-mIBG over 12 months. (B) Diagnostic scan done 18 months post-therapy shows no uptake of tracer in the liver metastases and low-grade uptake in the mesenteric mass essentially reflecting a good response to I-131-mIBG therapy

hormonal responses in 45%. Five patients were also reported to have had complete tumour and hormonal responses (16–58 months). However, the types of tumours in this review included a combination of metastatic phaeochromocytoma (66%) and paraganglioma (34%)[13]. Various other groups have also reported an overall tumour response (which includes partial tumour response or stabilization of the disease) in more than 50% of the patients[14,24–26].

Metastatic carcinoid tumours

Unlike patients with metastatic catecholamine-secreting tumours, experience with 131I-mIBG for carcinoid tumours is limited. A global experience of

Table 5.5 Summary of early and late side-effects/complications of radiolabelled mIBG and somatostatin analogues

^{131}I-mIBG	Nausea and vomiting 24–48 h Transient myelosuppression (4–6 weeks) Haematological effects (reported as an isolated thrombocytopenia) Rarely deterioration of renal function (observed in patients pretreated with chemotherapy) Serotonin release in carcinoid patients may cause flushing Hypothyroidism (if inadequate thyroid blockade) Persistent haematological effects (thrombocytopenia, myelosuppression)
^{90}Y-DOTA-Tyr^3)-Octreotide	Renal toxicity, thrombocytopenia and liver toxicity were reported in some patients and nausea and vomiting were observed in patients treated with amino acids. Transient myelosuppression One patient developed myelodysplastic syndrome
^{90}Y-DOTA-lanreotide (MAURITIUS)	No severe acute or chronic haematological toxicity, change in renal or liver function parameters caused by ^{90}Y-DOTA-lanreotide treatment were reported for patients in the MAURITIUS trial
^{177}Lu-TATE [DOTA^O-Tyr^3]	Haematological toxicity (leucocytopenia and thrombocytopenia) of grade 2 and 3 were observed in some Mild nausea, vomiting, and mild abdominal discomfort were present in some patients

the treatment of 52 patients was reported in 1994, where an objective tumour response was recorded in 15% and symptomatic responses in 65%[27]. However, recent studies are more encouraging. Safford *et al.*, treated 98 patients with metastatic carcinoid tumour, they reported symptomatic response in 35 patients (49%), hormonal response in 52 patients (53%), and a radiographic tumour response in 75 patients (75.5%)[28]. Five-year survival rate after treatment for the entire group of patients was 22%. There were 27 actual 5-year survivors, which is encouraging. It was observed that patients who had symptomatic response to ^{131}I-mIBG therapy demonstrated an increased median survival of 5.76 versus 2.09 years for patients who had no response or progression of symptoms. Taal *et al.* reported a long-term palliative effect in 60% of patients with metastatic carcinoid tumours treated with ^{131}I-mIBG[22,29]. Mukherjee *et al.* reported similar results with a subjective response in 73% of patients (11 of 18 patients)[24]. Pathirana *et al*, reported a subjective response rate of 83% of patients, following only one cycle of ^{131}I-mIBG[23].

Malignant medullary thyroid cancer

The worldwide cumulative experience reported in the last decade reported an objective tumour response in approximately 30% of patients and a symptomatic response in 50%[27,30,31]. Since then, further studies have been reported but the number of patients is very small[32–34].

5.5 **Peptides and radionuclide therapy**

Peptides are labelled with a variety of radionuclides for therapeutic applications in neuroendocrine tumours. Peptides are easy to synthesize, have fast clearance, rapid tissue penetration, and show high affinity for characteristic receptor molecules that are over expressed on malignant mammalian cells[35]. In general, peptides are less likely to be immunogenic than monoclonal antibodies.

The peptide that has attracted great interest as an imaging agent is SMS. SMS is a tetra-decapeptide that regulates the secretion of numerous hormones[36]. Receptors for SMS are expressed on a variety of human tumours and it is this property that has led to the use of SMS analogues for tumour imaging and therapy[9,35,37–39].

5.5.1 **Radiolabelled somatostatin analogue therapy**

SMS is a cyclic 14-amino acid peptide, which is widely distributed in the body and has multiple sites of action[40]. Most neuroendocrine tumours such as carcinoids, paragangliomas, phaeochromocytomas, and pancreatic-endocrine tumours express a high density of SMS receptors (SSR 1–5)[41–43]. Various types of SMS analogues, such as octreotide, lanreotide, and octreotate recognize the SMS receptors (especially SSR 2, SSR 5 and SSR 3) and bind to them with high affinity and specificity[9,44–47]. The half-life of the natural SMS is less than 2 minutes, which makes it less favourable for radionuclide therapy. SMS analogues with long half-life are commonly used in the medical management of carcinoid tumours[48–50].

Radiolabelled (^{111}In, ^{90}Y and ^{177}Lu) SMS analogues have been used for neuroendocrine tumour therapy (Table 5.6). The major drawback of ^{111}In is the short range of the therapeutic Auger electrons emitted and the relatively high renal dose from ^{111}In-DTPA^0]octreotide, thus this radiopharmaceutical is now out of favour. Most therapies are now carried out using ^{90}Y(Yttrium-90) and ^{177}Lu (Lutetium-177) radionuclides. DOTA (1,4,7,10-tetraazacyclododecane-1,4,7,10-tetra-acetic acid) is currently used as an ideal chelator since it is reported to form complexes, which are both thermodynamically and kinetically stable[51].

As part of the selection process (Table 5.7) all patients should have [^{111}In-DTPA^0]octreotide/pentetreotide scintigraphy (Octreoscan) (Fig. 5.3) or ^{68}Ga-Octreotate PET/CT scan prior to therapy. The tumour uptake should be at least as high as the uptake in the normal liver tissue[52].

Table 5.6 Summary of targeted therapy with radiolabelled somatostatin analogues

Radiopharmaceuticals	¹¹¹Indium-Pentetreotide	⁹⁰Yttrium-pentetreotide	⁹⁰Yttrium-lanreotide	¹⁷⁷Lutitium-octreotate
Type of radiation	Auger electrons	High-energy β-emitter (>1 mm)	High-energy β-emitter (>1 mm)	Low-energy β- and γ-emitter (<200 μm)
Half-life (t₁/₂)	67 hours	64 hours	64 hours	160.8 hours
Chelator	DTPA	DOTA	DOTA	DOTA
Dose	Up to 5 GBq/cycle	1–4.4 GBq/cycle	1.2 GBq/cycle	3.7–7.4 GBq/cycle
Amino acid co-infusion	No	Yes	No	Yes
Receptor affinity	Binds to SS receptor 2 and 5 with high affinity and to SS 3 with moderate affinity Does not bind to receptor 1 and 4	Binds to SS receptor 2 and 5 with high affinity and to SS 3 with moderate affinity Does not bind to receptor 1 and 4	Binds to SS receptors 2, 3, 4, and 5 with high affinity Binds to receptor 1 with lower affinity	Octreotate has ninefold higher affinities for the SS receptor 2
Advantages	Imaging can be performed	Better for large tumours	Better for large tumours	Imaging is feasible
Disadvantages	Short path length of Auger electrons Very few centres use ¹¹¹In-pentetreotide to treat patients	Quantitative imaging cannot be performed	Quantitative imaging cannot be performed	Optimal only for small tumours

Table 5.7 Radiolabelled somatostatin analogue therapy* (Kindly note all the above mentioned protocols are arbitrary and currently there are no strict guidelines)

Eligibility criteria and checklist prior therapy

1. Patients should have a biopsy proven, inoperable neuroendocrine tumour and have undergone conventional staging investigations (computed tomography/magnetic resonance imaging, biochemical markers)

2. ^{111}In-pentretreotide (octreoscan) positive tumours, documented by quantitative tracer scan

3. Ensure name, date of birth, and the hospital number is correct and make positive identification of the patient

4. Explain the procedure to the patient

5. Patients should receive both written and verbal information about the procedure and informed written consent must be obtained from the patient.

6. Careers should receive specific instruction in radiation safety precautions

Procedure/protocol:

Set up ^{90}Y-lanreotide/^{90}Y-Dotatoc trolleys

Give ^{90}Y-lanreotide(without amino acids)/^{90}Y-DOTATOC(with amino acids)

^{90}Y-Dotatoc: 500 ml of Hartman (Hepa 8% amino acid) solution is given 30 minutes before injecting the radiolabelled (^{90}Y-Dotatoc) somatostatin analogue. After intravenous injection of ^{90}Y-Dotatoc, an additional dose of 1500 ml of amino acids are infused over a period of 3–31/2 hours

^{90}Y-Lanreotide: 1.2 GBq infused over about 30 minutes 4–6 weeks apart

After care check renal and BM function every 2 weeks (normally get GP to do this and send results in until 8 weeks after last treatment

(Can give second set of treatment with a 6-month break maximum is six treatments)

^{90}Y-Octreotate: Start amino acids infusion (1 litre Viamin 18 or similar) at a rate of 1 litre per 4 hours or slower if vomiting occurs give 8 mg oral ondansetron and wait for 30 minutes

3–4 GBq of ^{90}Y-Octreotate is infused over 20–30 minutes. Continue amino acids till finished

Treatment can be repeated at 6–8 week period for three treatments only and no further treatments are currently recommended

Remove the trolley and administration kit from the room

Patient instruction and precautions

Check trolley and staff for contamination

Return the waste to the hot lab in nuclear medicine for disposal

Set up radiation protection procedures and appropriate signage on the door

Discharge patient home by 16–24 hours post-treatment

Check the room for contamination after sending the patient home

Decontaminate the room and make it available for next patient

Post therapy imaging:

^{90}Y imaging next day if useful and available

Follow up:

Tumour response assessment using conventional radiological or radionuclide methods

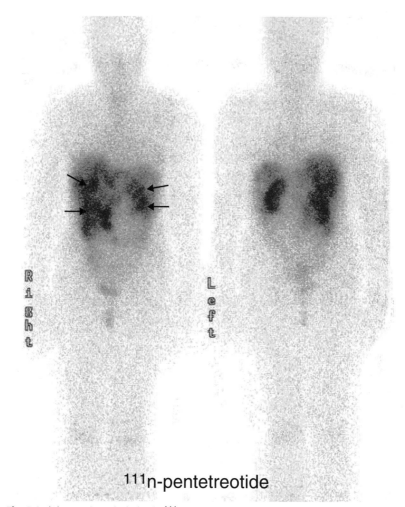

Fig. 5.3 (A) Anterior whole body ^{111}In-pentetreotide (Octreoscan) scan in a patient with neuroendocrine tumours, showing multiple somatostatin receptor positive metastases in the liver (arrows) (B) Posterior whole body view showing prominent tracer retention in kidneys.

As with ^{131}I-MIBG, there are no consensual published guidelines for [90]Y- or ^{177}Lu-labelled SMS analogues dose or dose schedules for palliative therapy. Most literature reports show dose ranges between 3.7–5.5 GBq of ^{90}Y and 3.7–7.4 GBq of ^{177}Lu labelled SMS analogues[53–57]. Several doses may be required to obtain an objective response and the treatment should not be repeated less than 4–6 weeks.

5.5.2 Clinical efficacies of radionuclide somatostatin analogue therapies

(^{90}Y-DOTA-Tyr^3)-Octreotide (^{90}Y-DOTATOC)

In the phase I/II studies, patients with neuroendocrine tumours were treated with four intravenous injections of ^{90}Y-DOTATOC. Dose escalation studies have revealed a dose of 5.18GBq as the maximum tolerable dose of ^{90}Y-DOTA-TOC per cycle[56,58,59]. As the kidneys with a significant element of binding excrete these radiopharmaceuticals, the dose to the kidneys should be limited to 27 Gy[60]. Renal protection is achieved with intravenous co-infusion of amino acid (Arginine and Lysine) using Hartmann-HEPA 8%)[6,54–56]. Assuming there are no toxicities the doses can be repeated at 6-week intervals.

In radiolabelled SMS analogue therapy, the radiation dose to the kidneys poses an important limit to the amount of radioactivity that can be administered safely. Renal function loss and even end-stage renal disease have been reported after therapy with ^{90}Y-DOTATOC[61,62]. The injected radiolabelled octreotide is efficiently reabsorbed by cells in the proximal tubule of the nephron, where a significant amount of activity is retained[63,64]. Other adverse effects include nausea and vomiting (grade I–II gastrointestinal toxicity) in 48% of patients[39,56,58,59]. Patients can develop grade II–III haematological toxicity[56,58,59]. Thrombocytopenia and liver toxicity have also been reported in some patients. In the long term, few patients developed myelodysplastic syndrome and leucopenia[60].

Summarizing the data and confirmed with from personal experience, improvement in clinical symptoms was observed in more than 60% of patients. An objective response was reported in 23% of the patients (WHO criteria), complete remission of disease has been reported in <5%, partial response in about 20%, stable disease in about 55% and progression in the remaining patients. These promising tumour responses after therapy are essentially similar to those found in other ^{90}Y-DOTATOC studies, despite differences in therapy regimens[55,57,60–66].

^{90}Y-DOTA-lanreotide

The structure of DOTA-lanreotide is different from DOTA-octreotide. The C-terminus DOTA-lanreotide has a ThrNH$_2$ and at the N-terminus, D-phe is replaced by a D-2 naphthylalanine[67]. This modification in the structure is reported to lower the kidney dose and co-infusion of amino acid is not required. However, dose to bone marrow, whole-body, liver, and intestine is higher. ^{90}Y-DOTA-lanreotide is a universal SMS receptor subtype ligand that binds all the five-SMS receptor types[68]. ^{90}Y-DOTA-lanreotide binds with high affinity to SMS receptors 2–5 and intermediate affinity for receptor 1[68].

In the *MAURITIUS* (Multicenter Analysis of a Universal Receptor Imaging and Treatment Initiative, a European Study) trial cumulative treatment doses up to 8.5 GBq ^{90}Y-DOTA-lanreotide were given as a short-term intravenous infusion. Results in 154 patients showed partial response in 14% (22 of 154) and stable tumour disease in 41% (63 of 154) of patients[69]. No acute or chronic toxic events were reported[69].

^{177}Lu-TATE [DOTA^0-Tyr^3]-octreotide

^{177}Lu-DOTATATE is a more recent development, which shows great promise[70,71]. This seems to show relatively high tumour uptake of all tested octreotide analogues so far, not only in rats but also in patients with neuroendocrine tumours[72]. ^{177}Lu-DOTATATE, has twice as high affinity as ^{90}Y-DOTATOC, gives a greater tumour-to-kidney ratio, thereby gives a wider therapeutic window for therapy[71]. The SMS analogue [DOTA^0,Tyr^3] octreotate has a ninefold higher affinity for the SMS receptor subtype 2 compared with [DOTA^0,Tyr^3]octreotide *in vitro*[73,74] ^{177}Lu would be optimal for small tumours and post-therapy imaging is also feasible. The main strength of ^{177}Lu-octreotate is the ability to carry out whole body imaging post-therapy. This helps to confirm the delivery of radionuclide to target sites and calculate the radiation dose delivered to tumour sites.

In a preliminary report, Kwekkeboom *et al.*, in their first 35 patients treated with ^{177}Lu-octreotate, they showed partial response in significant number of patients[71]. In a more recent update[75] of this treatment, 131 patients were treated with cumulative doses of 22.2–29.6 GBq (600–800 mCi) of ^{177}Lu-octreotate. Of the 125 evaluable patients complete remission was reported in three patients, partial remission in 32 patients, minor response in 24 patients, stable disease in 44 patients and progressive disease in 22 patients). The median time to progression was more than 36 months, which compares favourably with chemotherapy. Results were better in patients with a limited tumour load.

Nausea and vomiting (WHO toxicity Grade 1–2) within the first 24 hours after the administration were present in 31% and 14% of the administrations, respectively. Mild abdominal pain was noticed by 12% of the patients, especially those with liver enlargement. Increased hair loss (WHO toxicity grade 1) was noticed by 64% of the patients; hair re-growth occurred within 3 months after the last administration. Serious side-effects that were potentially treatment related were found in only two patients. One patient had renal insufficiency and another patient developed hepatorenal syndrome. However, Creatinine clearance did not change significantly in the other patients, as use of amino acid co-infusion limited the estimated cumulative dose to the kidneys to 23 Gy or less[75].

5.6 **Recent advances and future**

5.6.1 **Combination therapy with ^{90}Y-labelled and ^{177}Lu somatostatin analogues**

Clinical trials of ^{90}Y-labelled and ^{177}Lu SMS analogues have demonstrated the use of these compounds in targeted radionuclide therapy[74]. However, these radiolabelled compounds differ in their physical properties (half-life, energy type, and path length)[74]. In patients with large/bulky tumours, poorly vascularized and heterogeneous tumour setting, treatment with ^{90}Y-labelled compounds is preferable. However, in patients with smaller tumours, therapy with ^{177}Lu SMS analogues is preferable. The combination of these two compounds could improve the clinical therapeutic outcome in patients treated with radiolabelled SMS analogues. In a rat model, the antitumour effects of 50% ^{90}Y- and ^{177}Lu-labelled SMS analogues were superior to those animals treated with either ^{90}Y or ^{177}Lu SMS analogues alone[74]. The combination of repeated administration of these compounds, such as initial administration with ^{90}Y-labelled analogues for larger tumours, followed by ^{177}Lu analogues to treat smaller tumour is an option being tested in clinical trials and results are awaited[74]. Such an approach requires caution as individually both these compounds have advantages and disadvantages, based on numerous factors.

5.7 **Radioembolization/intra-arterial ^{90}Y-Lanreotide therapy**

The possible risk of bone marrow toxicity with repeated use of ^{90}Y-SMS analogue therapy led investigators to use intra-arterial infusion of radiolabelled SMS analogues. Neuroendocrine tumours tend to metastasize to the liver, where they receive most of their blood supply from the hepatic artery. Thus, hepatic administration of beta-emitting radionuclides presents an attractive approach to deliver therapeutic focal irradiation[76,77]. The technique involves identification of the right and left hepatic artery and its catheterization. Once this has been achieved 1.2 GBq of ^{90}Y-SMS analogue is infused in about 5 minutes using a 5F catheter into the hepatic artery[78]. Many groups are also investigating the role of intra-arterial radiolabelled micro spheres. However, the results of these studies are awaited. Post-therapy bremmstrahlung imaging can be performed (if available) to assess localization[78] (Figs 5.4 and 5.5).

5.8 **Medical management**

Medical management of neuroendocrine tumours involves SMS analogues, IFN-α, and chemotherapy[5,79].

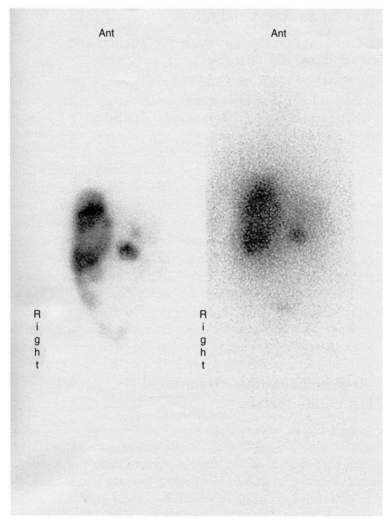

Fig. 5.4 (A) Anterior whole body ^{111}In-pentetreotide (Octreoscan) diagnostic scan showing multiple somatostatin receptor positive metastases. (B) Post-therapy bremmstrahlung imaging following intravenous ^{90}Y-octreotate administration.

5.8.1 **Somatostatin analogues**

Octreotide, a SMS analogue, is reported to be the best therapy for controlling symptoms and it reduces flushing and diarrhoea in more than 70% and 60% of patients respectively[80]. Octreotide is also reported to have some inhibitory effect on tumour growth[81]. Initially octreotide should be given in small doses and may be gradually increased. Some patients may require

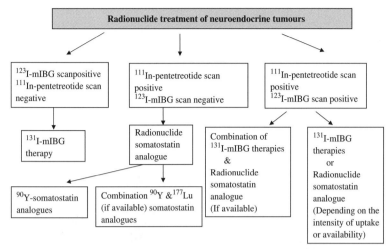

Fig. 5.5 Proposed treatment algorithm for the treatment of neuroendocrine tumours.

higher doses. However, Several patients have become resistant to high-dose octreotide given over an extended period due to an escape effect whereby even the highest doses do not have any benefit[4]. Currently, lanreotide also SMS analogue with a slow-release formulation is available and is given as an intramuscular injection. Lanreotide in addition to the convenience of its use, it is also shown to be as effective as octreotide in controlling symptoms and may have some antitumour activity[4,50,77,82,83].

5.8.2 **Chemotherapy**

Using a single chemotherapeutic agent has not been encouraging with response rate of less than 10%[5]. Reports suggest that a combination of streptozotocin with doxorubicin or 5-fluorouracil has generated response rates between 0 and 30%[84–86]. The role of chemotherapy is confined predominantly to patients with metastatic disease or anaplastic neuroendocrine tumours who are symptomatic and unresponsive to other therapies[5,79]. A response rate of up to 65% has been reported when a combination of cisplatin and etoposide is used in patients with anaplastic neuroendocrine tumours[87].

5.8.3 **Interferon-α**

IFN-α is used in treatment of neuroendocrine (carcinoids) tumours, because it has an ability to stimulate natural killer function and also controls symptoms, secretion of hormones and tumour growth[5,88]. Oberg and Eriksson have reported a biochemical response in 50%, stabilization in 35%, and significant tumour reduction in 15% of patients[89]. The mean duration of response was 32 months[5]. IFN-α has not gained popularity because of side-effects like chronic fatigue syndrome, anaemia, flu-like symptoms, and altered liver enzymes and most of these are dose dependent[5].

5.9 Hepatic artery chemoembolization

Patients with advanced metastatic carcinoid tumours who have disease progression are left with few treatment options. Hepatic artery chemoembolization may play a role in palliating these patients' symptoms[76]. Preliminary studies have shown that complications are low and, if the tumour pattern is nodular with some hypervascularity, beneficial results may develop both clinically and in terms of tumour burden[21,90].

Symptomatic flushing as well as 5-hydroxyindoleacetic acid concentrations decreases in up to 80% of patients[83]. Many studies have also shown regression in tumour size and some have reported an increase in median survival of up to 2 years[91].

5.10 Radiotherapy for neuroendocrine tumours

Radiotherapy is useful in regionally advanced or metastatic disease. Carcinoid tumours and islet cell tumours grow in a region with complex anatomy, containing various sensitive tissues and organs such as the kidneys, liver, stomach, small intestine, and the spinal cord[92]. Adequate care has to be taken not to exceed the tolerance doses for irradiation of these sensitive organs[92]. Exceeding these doses can result in complications like tissue necrosis, ulceration, perforation, and neurological effects. However, radiation therapy has a potential to arrest tumour growth and hormone secretion. Radiotherapy also causes pain relief and improvement of compression symptoms caused by bone and spinal metastases[92].

5.11 Conclusions

The last decade has seen major expansion in the role of radiolabelled mIBG and SMS analogues in treating NETs with reasonable success, and further scope of improvement. Protocols evaluating the combination of chemotherapy and radionuclide therapy are being tested, as it is shown that neither radiolabelled mIBG or SMS analogues identify all tumour sites, therefore some tumour cells will always escape. Other novel radiopharmaceuticals are also being tested and require balancing the benefits (clinical response to radionuclide therapy) and risks (radio toxicity) preferably on an individualized basis.

More data are required to assess the full clinical impact of these therapeutic modalities. Finally, every patient with NET should ideally receive 'tailor-made' therapy based on his or her particular tumour biology profile.

References

1. Gilligan CJ, Lawton GP, Tang LH, West AB and Modlin IM (1995). Gastric carcinoid tumors: the biology and therapy of an enigmatic and controversial lesion. *American Journal of Gastroenterology* **90**: 338–53.

2. Taal BG, Visser O (2004). Epidemiology of neuroendocrine tumours. *Neuroendocrinology* **80**: (Suppl. 1): 3–7.

3. Newton JN, Swerdlow AJ, dos Santos Silva IM, *et al.* (1994). The epidemiology of carcinoid tumours in England and Scotland. *British Journal of Cancer* **70**: 939–42.

4. Caplin ME, Buscombe JR, Hilson AJ, Jones AL, Watkinson AF, Burroughs AK (1998). Carcinoid tumour. *Lancet* **352**: 799–805.

5. Öberg, K (2005) Neuroendocrine tumors of the gastrointestinal tract: recent advances in molecular genetics, diagnosis, and treatment. *Current Opinion in Oncology* **17(4)**: 386–91.

6. Waldherr C, Pless M, Maecke HR, *et al.* (2002). Tumor response and clinical benefit in neuroendocrine tumors after 7.4 GBq ^{90}Y-DOTATOC. *Journal of Nuclear Medicine* **43**: 610–16.

7. Vucina J, Han R (2001). Use of radionuclides in therapy. *Medicinski Pregled* **54**: 245–50.

8. Ackery D (1998). Principles of radionuclide therapy. In Murray IPC, Ell PJ (ed.), *Nuclear medicine in clinical diagnosis and treatment*, Vol. 2, pp. 1039–42. New York: Churchill Livingstone.

9. Lamberts SWJ, Krenning EP, Reubi JC (1991). The role of somatostatin and its analogs in the diagnosis and treatment of tumours. *Endocrine Reviews* **12**: 450–82.

10. Le Rest C, Bomanji JB, Costa DC, Townsend CE, Visvikis D, Ell PJ (2001). Functional imaging of metastatic neuroendocrine tumours. *European Journal of Nuclear Medicine* **28**: 478–482.

11. Sisson JC, Shapiro B, Beierwaltes WH, *et al.* (1984). Radiopharmaceutical treatment of malignant pheochromocytoma. *Journal of Nuclear Medicine* **25(2)**: 197–206.

12. Hoefnagel CA, Voute PA, de Kraker J, Marcuse HR (1987).Radionuclide diagnosis and therapy of neural crest tumors using iodine-131 metaiodobenzylguanidine. *Journal of Nuclear Medicine* **28(3)**: 308–14.

13. Loh KC, Fitzgerald PA, Matthay KK, Yeo PP, Price DC (1997). The treatment of malignant pheochromocytoma with iodine-131 metaiodobenzylguanidine (131I-MIBG): a comprehensive review of 116 reported patients. *Journal of Endocrinological Investigation* **20**: 648–58.

14. Bomanji JB, Wong W, Gaze MN, *et al.* (2003). Treatment of neuroendocrine tumours in adults with 131I-MIBG therapy. *Clinical Oncology* **15**: 193–8.

15. Guidelines for 131I-meta Iodo Benzylguanidine Therapy (2002) (EANM Radionuclide Therapy Committee guidelines), www.eanm.org

16. Solanki KK, Bomanji JB, Moyes J, Mather SJ, Trainer PJ, Britton KE (1992). A pharmacological guide to medicines which interfere with the biodistribution of radiolabelled meta-iodobenzylguanidine (MIBG). *Nuclear Medicine Communications* **13(7)**: 513–21.

17. Solanki KK, Bomanji JB, Waddington WA, Ell PJ (2004). Thyroid blocking policy: Revisited. *Nuclear Medicine Communications* 25(11): 1071–6.

18. Hoefnagel CA, Lewington VJ (2004) MIBG therapy. In: Ell PJ, Gambhir SS (eds), *Nuclear medicine in clinical diagnosis and treatment*, Vol. 1, pp. 445–557. New York: Churchill Livingstone.

19. Bomanji J, Hawkins LA, Ur E, Grossman A, Foley R, Granowska M, Besser GM, Britton KE (1992). Treatment of malignant phaeochromocytoma, paraganglioma and carcinoid tumours with I-131 metaiodobenzylguanidine. *Nuclear Medicine Communications*, 14: 856–861.

20. Prvulovich EM, Stein RC, Bomanji JB, Ledermann JA, Taylor I, Ell PJ (1998). Iodine-131-MIBG therapy of a patient with carcinoid liver metastases. *Journal of Nuclear Medicine* 39: 1743–5.

21. Kaltsas G, Rockall A, Papadogias D, Reznek R, Grossman AB (2004). Recent advances in radiological and radionuclide imaging and therapy of neuroendocrine tumours *European Journal of Endocrinology* 15b1: 15–27.

22. Taal BG, Hoefnagel CA, Valdes Olmos RA, Boot H, Beijnen JH(1996) Palliative effect of metaiodobenzylguanidine in metastatic carcinoid tumors. *Journal of Clinical Oncology* 14: 1829–38.

23. Pathirana AA, Vinjamuri S, Byrne C, Ghaneh P, Vora J, Poston GJ (2001). (131)I-MIBG radionuclide therapy is safe and cost-effective in the control of symptoms of the carcinoid syndrome. *European Journal of Surgical Oncology* 27: 404–8.

24. Mukherjee JJ, Kaltsas GA, Islam N (2001). Treatment of metastatic carcinoid tumours, phaeochromocytoma, paraganglioma and medullary carcinoma of the thyroid with (131)I-metaiodobenzylguanidine [(131)I-mIBG]. *Clinical Endocrinology* 55: 47–60.

25. Kaltsas G, Mukherjee JJ, Foley R, Britton K, Grossman A (2003). Treatment of metastatic pheochromocytoma and paraganglioma with 131I-meta-iodobenzylguanidine (MIBG). *Endocrinologist* 13: 1–13.

26. Ackery DM, Troncone L (1991). Session on the role of [131I]metaiodobenzylguanidine in the treatment of malignant phaeochromocytoma. Chairmen's report. *Journal Nuclear Biology and Medicine* 35: 318–20.

27. Hoefnagel CA (1994). Metaiodobenzylguanidine and somatostatin in oncology: role in the management of neural crest tumours. *European Journal of Nuclear Medicine* 21: 561–81.

28. Safford SD, Coleman RE, Gockerman JP (2004). Iodine-131 metaiodobenzylguanidine treatment for metastatic carcinoid. Results in 98 patients. *Cancer* 101: 1987–93.

29. Taal BG, Hoefnagel C, Boot H, Valdes OR, Rutgers M (2000). Improved effect of 131I-MIBG treatment by predosing with non-radiolabeled MIBG in carcinoid patients, and studies in xenografted mice. *Annals of Oncology* 11: 1437–43.

30. Hoefnagel CA, Delprat CC, Valdes Olmos RA (1991). Role of [131I]metaiodobenzylguanidine therapy in medullary thyroid carcinoma. *Journal of Nuclear and Biological Medicine* 35: 334–6.

31. Troncone L, Rufini V, Maussier M, *et al.* (1991). The role of [131I]metaiodobenzylguanidine in the treatment of medullary thyroid carcinoma: results in five cases. *Journal of Nuclear and Biological Medicine* 35: 327–31.

32. Castellani MR, Alessi A, Savelli G, Bombardieri E (2004).The role of radionuclide therapy in medullary thyroid cancer. *Tumori* **89**: 560–2.

33. Chatal JF, Le Bodic MF, Kraeber-Bodere F, Rousseau C, Resche I (2000). Nuclear medicine applications for neuroendocrine tumors. *World Journal of Surgery* **24**: 1285–9.

34. Rufini V, Salvatori M, Garganese MC, *et al.* (2000). Role of nuclear medicine in the diagnosis and therapy of medullary thyroid carcinoma. *Rays* **25**: 273–82.

35. Weiner RE, Thakur ML (2001). Radiolabeled peptides in diagnosis and therapy. *Seminars in Nuclear Medicine* **31**(4): 296–311.

36. Bruns C, Raulf F, Hoyer D, Schloos J, Luebbert H, Weckbecker G (1996). Binding properties of somatostatin receptor subtypes. *Metabolism: Clinical and Experimental* **45**: 17–20.

37. Lamberts SWJ (1988). The role of somatostatin in the regulation of anterior pituitary hormone secretion and the use of its analogues in the treatment of human pituitary tumors. *Endocrine Reviews* **9**: 417–36.

38. Thakur ML, Kolan H, Li J, *et al.* (1997). Radiolabeled somatostatin analogues in prostate cancer. *Nuclear Biology and Medicine* **24**: 105–13.

39. de Jong M, Breeman WA, Bernard HF, *et al.* (1999). Therapy of neuroendocrine tumor with radiolabeled somatostatin analogues. *Quarterly Journal of Nuclear Medicine* **43**: 356–66.

40. Reubi JC, Laissue J, Waser B, *et al.* (1994). Expression of somatostatin receptors in normal, inflamed and neoplastic human gastrointestinal tissues. *Annals of the New York Academy of Sciences* **733**: 122–37.

41. Virgolini I, Pangerl T, Bischof C, Smith-Jones P, Peck-Radosavljevic M (1997). Somatostatin receptor subtype expression in human tissues: a prediction for diagnosis and treatment of Cancer. *European Journal of Clinical Investigation* **27**: 645–7.

42. Reubi JC, Kvols L, Krenning E, Lamberts SW (1990). Distribution of somatostatin receptors in normal and tumor tissue. *Metabolism* **39**: 78–81.

43. Reubi JC, Laissue J, Krenning E, Lamberts SW (1992). Somatostatin receptors in human cancer: incidence, characteristics, functional correlates and clinical implications. *Journal of Steroid Biochemistry and Molecular Biology* **43**: 27–35.

44. Reubi JC, Lamberts SW, Maurer R (1988). Somatostatin receptors in normal and tumoral tissue. *Hormone Research* **29**: 65–9.

45. Reubi JC, Kvols LK, Waser B, *et al.* (1990). Detection of somatostatin receptors in surgical and percutaneous needle biopsy samples of carcinoids and islet cell carcinomas. *Cancer Research* **50**: 5969–77.

46. Papotti M, Macri L, Bussolati G, Reubi JC (1989). Correlative study on neuro-endocrine differentiation and presence of somatostatin receptors in breast carcinomas. *International Journal of Cancer* **43**: 365–9.

47. Hofland LJ, van Hagen PM, Lamberts SW (1999). Functional role of somatostatin receptors in neuroendocrine and immune cells. *Annals of Medicine* **31**: 23–7.

48. Faiss S, Scherubl H, Riecken EO, Wiedenmann B (1996). Drug therapy in metastatic neuroendocrine tumors of the gastroenteropancreatic system. *Recent Results in Cancer Research* **142**: 193–207.

49. Ruszniewski P, Ducreux M, Chayvialle JA, *et al.* (1996). Treatment of the carcinoid syndrome with long acting somatostatin analogue lanreotide: a prospective study in 39 patients. *Gut* **39**: 279–83.

50. Oberg K (1998). Advances in chemotherapy and biotherapy of endocrine tumors. *Current Opinion in Oncology* **10**: 58–65.

51. Stolz B, Weckbecker G, Smith-Jones PM, Albert R, Raulf F, Bruns C (1998). The somatostatin receptor targeted radiotherapeutic [90Y-DTPA-Dphe1,Tyr3]octreotide (90Y-SMT 487) eradicates experimental rat pancreatic CA 20948 tumours. *European Journal of Nuclear Medicine* **25**; 668–74.

52. Lewington VJ (2003). Targeted radionuclide therapy for neuroendocrine tumours *Endocrine-Related Cancer* **10**: 497–501.

53. Kwekkeboom D, Krenning EP, de Jong M (2000). Peptide receptor imaging and therapy.*Journal of Nuclear Medicine* **41**: 1704–13.

54. Waldherr C, Pless M, Maecke HR, Haldemann A, Mueller-Brand J (2001). The clinical value of [90Y-DOTA]-D-Phe1-Tyr3-octreotide (90Y-DOTATOC) in the treatment of neuroendocrine tumours: a clinical phase II study. *Annals of Oncology* **12**: 941–5.

55. Bodei L, Cremonesi M, Zoboli S, *et al.* (2003) Receptor mediated radiotherapy with 90Y-DOTATOC in association with amino acid infusion; a phase I study. *European Journal of Nuclear Medicine* **30**: 207–16.

56. Paganelli G, Zoboli S, Cremonesi M, Macke HR, Chinol M (1999). Receptor-mediated radionuclide therapy with 90Y-DOTA-D-Phe1-Tyr3-Octreotide: preliminary report in cancer patients. *Cancer Biotherapy and Radiopharmaceutics* **14**: 477–83.

57. Valkema R, Jamar F, Bakker WH, *et al.* (2001). Safety and efficacy of [Y-90-DOTA, Tyr(3)]octreotide (Y-90-SMT487; OCTREOTHER™) peptide receptor radionuclide therapy (PRRT): preliminary results of a phase-1 study. *European Journal of Nuclear Medicine* **28**: 1025. (abstract)

58. Paganelli G, Zoboli S, Cremonesi M (2001). Receptor-mediated radiotherapy with 90Y-DOTA-D-Phe1-Tyr3-octreotide. *European Journal of Nuclear Medicine* **28**: 426–34.

59. Cremonesi M, Ferrari M, Zoboli S (1999). Biokinetics and dosimetry in patients administered with (111)In-DOTA-Tyr(3)-octreotide: implications for internal radiotherapy with (90)Y-DOTATOC. *European Journal of Nuclear Medicine* **26**: 877–86.

60. Valkemma R, Jamar F, Jonard P *et al.* (2000). Targeted radiotherapy with 90Y-DOTA-Tyr3-octreotide (90Y-SMT487; Octreother TM), a phase I study. *Journal of Nuclear Medicine* **41**(Suppl.): 111. (abstract)

61. Otte A, Herrmann R, Heppeler A, *et al.* (1999). Yttrium-90 DOTATOC: first clinical results. *European Journal of Nuclear Medicine* **26:** 1439–47.

62. Cybulla M, Weiner SM, Otte A (2001). End-stage renal disease after treatment with ^{90}Y-DOTATOC. *European Journal of Nuclear Medicine* **28**: 1552–4.

63. Christensen EI, Nielsen S (1991). Structural and functional features of protein handling in the kidney proximal tubule. *Seminars in Nephrology* **11**: 414–39.

64. de Jong M, Rolleman EJ, Bernard BF, *et al.* (1996). Inhibition of renal uptake of indium-111-DTPA-octreotide in vivo. *Journal of Nuclear Medicine* **37:** 1388–92.

65. Buscombe JR, Caplin ME, Hilson AJ (2003). Long-term efficacy of high activity 111In-pentetreotide therapy in patients with disseminated neuroendocrine tumors. *Journal of Nuclear Medicine* **44**: 1–6.

66. Chinol M, Bodei L, Cremonesi M, Paganelli G (2002). Receptor-mediated radiotherapy with Y-DOTA-DPhe-Tyr-octreotide: the experience of the European Institute of Oncology Group. *Seminars in Nuclear Medicine* **32**: 141–7.

67. Giusti M, Ciccarelli E, Dallabonzana D (1997). Clinical results of long term slow release lanreotide treatment of acromegaly. *European Journal of Clinical Investigation* **27**: 277–84.

68. Smith-Jones PM, Bischof C, Leimer M, *et al.* (1999). DOTA-Lanreotide: a novel somatostatin analog for tumor diagnosis and therapy. *Endocrinology* **140**: 5136–48.

69. Virgolini I, Britton K, Buscombe J, Moncayo R, Paganelli G, Riva P (2002). In- and Y-DOTA-lanreotide: results and implications of the MAURITIUS trial. *Seminars in Nuclear Medicine* **3**: 148–55.

70. Kwekkeboom DJ, Bakker WH, Kooij PP, *et al.* (2001). [177Lu-DOTAOTyr3]octreotate: comparison with [111In-DTPAo]octreotide in patients. *European Journal of Nuclear Medicine* **28**: 1319–25.

71. Kwekkeboom DJ, Bakker WH, Kam BL, *et al.* (2003). Treatment of patients with gastro-entero-pancreatic (GEP) tumours with the novel radiolabelled somatostatin analogue [177Lu-DOTA^0: Tyr^3]octreotate. *European Journal of Nuclear Medicine and Molecular Imaging* **30**: 417–22.

72. de Jong M, Breeman WA, Bernard BF (2001). [177Lu-DOTA(0),Tyr3] octreotate for somatostatin receptor-targeted radionuclide therapy. *International Journal of Cancer* **92**: 628–33.

73. Reubi JC, Schar JC, Waser B, *et al.* (2000) Affinity profiles for human somatostatin receptor subtypes SST1-SST5 of somatostatin radiotracers selected for scintigraphic and radiotherapeutic use. *European Journal of Nuclear Medicine* **27**: 273–82.

74. de Jong M Breeman WAValkema R Bernard BF Krenning EP (2005) Combination radionuclide therapy using 177Lu- and 90Y-labeled somatostatin analogs. *Journal of Nuclear Medicine* **46**: 13–17S.

75. Kwekkeboom DJ, Teunissen JJ, Bakker WH, *et al.* (2005) Radiolabeled somatostatin analog [177Lu-DOTA0, Tyr3]octreotate in patients with endocrine gastroenteropancreatic tumors. *Journal of Clinical Oncology* **23**: 2754–62.

76. Drougas JG, Anthony LB, Blair TK *et al.* (1998). Hepatic artery chemoembolization for management of patients with advanced metastatic carcinoid tumors. *American Journal of Surgery* **175**: 408–12.

77. Astruc B, Marbach P, Bouterfa H (2005). Long-acting octreotide and prolonged-release lanreotide formulations have different pharmacokinetic profiles. *Journal of Clinical Pharmacology* **45**: 836–44.

78. Gnanasegaran G, Buscombe JR, O'Rourke E, Caplin ME, Purfield D, Hilson AJW (2005). Brehmsstrahlung imaging after intra-arterial ^{90}Y-lanreotide-radionuclide therapy for carcinoid liver metastases. *Nuclear Medicine Communications* **26**: 271–95.

79. Plöckinger U, Rindi G, Arnold R, Eriksson B, Krenning EP, de Herder WW, Goede A, Caplin M, Öberg K, Reubi JC, Nilsson O, Delle Fave G, Ruszniewski P, Ahlman H, Wiedenmann B (2004): Guidelines for the diagnosis and treatment of neuroendocrine gastrointestinal tumours. *Neuroendocrinology* **80**: 394–424.

80. Le Treut PY, Delpero JR, Dousset B *et al.* (1997). Results of liver transplantation in the treatment of metastatic neuroendocrine tumours. *Annals of Surgery* **225**: 335–64.

81. Arnold R, Frank M, Kajdan U (1995). Management of gastroenteropancreatic endocrine tumours: the place of somatostatin analogues. *Digestion* **55**: 107–13.

82. Norton JA (1994). Surgical management of carcinoid tumors: role of debulking and surgery for patients with advanced disease. *Digestion* **55**: 98–103.

83. Moertel CG, Johnson CM, McKusick MA, *et al.* (1994). The management of patients with advanced carcinoid tumours and islet cell carcinomas. *Annals of Internal Medicine* **120:** 302–9.

84. Moertel CG (1983). Treatment of the carcinoid tumor and the malignant carcinoid syndrome. *Journal of Clinical Oncology* **1:** 727–40.

85. Moertel CG, Hanley JA (1979). Combination chemotherapy trials in metastatic carcinoid tumor and the malignant carcinoid syndrome. *Cancer Clinical Trials* **2:** 327–33.

86. Norheim I, Öberg K, Alm G (1989). Treatment of malignant carcinoid tumors: a randomized controlled study of streptozocin plus 5-FU and human leukocyte interferon. *European Journal of Cancer and Clinical Oncology* **25:** 1475–9.

87. Moertel CG, Kvols LK, O'Connell MJ, *et al.* (1991). Treatment of neuro-endocrine carcinomas with combined etoposide and cisplatin. Evidence of major therapeutic activity in the anaplastic variants of these neoplasms. *Cancer* **68:** 227–32.

88. Öberg K, Funa K, Alm G (1983). Effects of leukocyte interferon upon clinical symptoms and hormone levels in patients with midgut carcinoid tumors and the carcinoid syndrome. *New England Journal of Medicine* **309:** 129–33.

89. Ö berg K, Eriksson B (1991). The role of interferons in the management of carcinoid tumors. *Acta Oncologica* **30:** 519–22.

90. Andrews JC, Walker SC, Ackermann RJ, Cotton LA, Ensminger WD, Shapiro B (1994). Hepatic radioembolization with yttrium-90 containing glass microspheres: preliminary results and clinical follow-up. *Journal of Nuclear Medicine* **35:** 1637–1644.

91. Mitty HA, Warner RR, Newman LH, Train JS, Parnes IH (1999). Control of carcinoid syndrome with hepatic artery embolization. *Radiology* **155:** 623–6.

92. Kiming BN (1994). Radiotherapy for gastroenteropancratic neuroendocrine tumours. Betram Weidman, Larry K Kvols, Rudlf Arnold, Ernst-Otto Riecken. In: *Molecular and cell biological aspects of gastroenteropancreatic neuroendocrine tumour disease. Annals of the New York Academy of Sciences* **733:** 488–495.

Chapter 6

Radioisotope therapy for metastatic bone disease

Peter Hoskin

6.1 Background to use

Bone metastasis are a common problem in the management of advanced malignancy being features of the common cancers, including breast cancer, prostate cancer, and lung cancer, which account for the majority of patients with symptomatic disease. The use of radioisotopes in bone metastases has focused predominantly upon patients with prostate cancer, although limited work in breast cancer has been undertaken with equal success. The principle of their use is to deliver targeted short-range radiation to sites of bone metastases using intravenous administration of a bone seeking radioisotope. The ideal agent will be specific for sites of bone damage secondary to metastatic invasion having predominantly beta emission depositing short-range radiation by decay to a stable solid daughter product. A small amount of low-energy gamma emission has some advantage in enabling imaging of the isotope distribution but the disadvantage of increased external radiation and therefore a requirement for more stringent radioprotection. The isotopes that have been used in this setting are phosphorus (^{32}P), strontium (^{89}Sr), samarium (^{153}Sm), and rhenium (^{186}Re and ^{189}Re). Other isotopes, which are currently under investigation, include tin (^{117}Sn) and radium (^{223}Ra), which is a pure alpha particle emitter[1,2]. Their radiation emissions and range are shown in Table 6.1.

There are three main mechanisms by which radioisotopes are concentrated at sites of bone metastasis:

1. Using an element that normal physiology will concentrate in bone at a site of remineralization. This relies on the fact that virtually all bone metastasis will have an element of osteoblastic response to the osteoclastic bone destruction provoked by the malignant cells. The osteoblastic response results in remineralization as a result of which certain chemicals, in particular calcium and phosphate, will be preferentially taken up at

Table 6.1 Isotopes in use for treatment of metastatic bone pain

	Therapeutic Formulation	Radiation	Half life	Range
Phosphorus	^{32}P PO$_4$	β	14.3 days	8 mm
Strontium	^{89}SrCl$_2$	β	50.5 days	6.7 mm
Samarium	^{153}SmEDTMP	β + γ	47 hours	3.4 mm
Rhenium	^{188}ReEDTP	β + γ	40 hours	10 mm
	^{186}ReEDTP	β + γ	16.5 hours	4.7 mm
Tin	^{117}SnDTPA	β + γ	13.6 days	<1 mm
Radium	^{223}RaCl	α	11.4 days	100 μm

those sites in the bone. This is the principle of a diagnostic isotope bone scan and has been used successfully for targeting therapeutic isotopes also. The two principal isotopes that have been used in this way are phosphorous (^{32}P) and strontium (^{89}Sr).

2. Incorporating the radioactive isotope in a complex molecule that is itself selectively taken up at sites of bone repair. The two examples in clinical use are samarium (^{153}Sm), which is presented in the complex Sm-EDTMP (ethylene diamine tetraline tetramethyline phosphonic acid), shown in Fig. 6.1, and rhenium [^{188}Re], which is presented in the complex Re-HEDP [1-1-hydroethylidene diphosphate]. There are two rhenium isotopes used, ^{186}Re and ^{188}Re. HEDP is in fact probably concentrated in bone by an osteoclast-dependent mechanism rather than an osteoblast dependent mechanism forming hydroxide bridges during hydrolysis of hydroxy apatite crystals.

3. Tumour-specific uptake. This is seen with metastases from thyroid cancer, which will take up ^{131}I, and neuroendocrine tumours, which will concentrate MIBG. These indications are discussed in Chapters 4 and 5 respectively and will not be considered further here.

Widespread uptake of radioactive chemicals at sites of bone metastases can result in a significant dose of radiation to the bone marrow. This was particularly prominent in the use of ^{32}P and one of the principal reasons for its use falling out of favour. Bone marrow suppression remains the dose-limiting toxicity for the modern isotopes strontium, samarium, and rhenium, upon which their administered doses are defined. The extent of bone marrow effect will depend upon the distribution and extent of metastases and the radiation quality; the range of the beta particles from strontium is up to

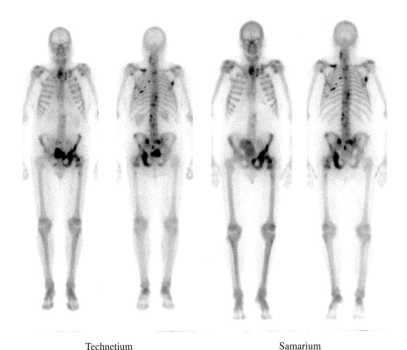

Technetium Samarium

Fig. 6.1 Samarium uptake in bone metastases demonstrated on gamma camera pictures alongside diagnostic technetium images (courtesy of Dr C. Hoefnagel, the Netherlands Cancer Institute).

7 mm, which may have a greater effect than the beta radiation from samarium having only a 3 mm range.

Clearance of these isotopes is predominantly renal and therefore accumulation in renal failure is to be expected resulting in prolonged bone marrow suppression. This is therefore a relative contraindication to their use.

6.2 Clinical indications

6.2.1 Therapeutic for palliation of metastatic bone pain

The principal indication for radioisotopes in metastatic bone pain is for the palliation of pain. Typically, they are used for patients who are no longer responsive to other systemic agents such as chemotherapy and hormone therapy who have several sites of bone pain or the typical clinical picture of pain flitting from one site to another. The role of radioisotopes for localized bone pain is less established and most patients will receive external beam radiotherapy for this, although it has been suggested that additional prophylaxis at other sites may be achieved[4] (see below).

Currently in the UK strontium is licensed for use in prostate cancer alone, although there are studies that have shown its efficacy in breast cancer patients. Samarium has wider licensed indications, including breast and prostate cancer.

6.2.2 Radical treatment

Radioisotopes are also under evaluation in research programmes to explore their role in ablating micrometastases and enabling longer-term control of established bone metastasis with a potential for not only reducing morbidity but also prolonging survival. Two particular initiatives have been published with interesting results.

The first of these has been to explore the use of strontium in combination with chemotherapy. In hormone refractory prostate cancer improved responses have been shown by combining strontium with cisplatin, carboplatin, doxorubicin[5,6] and also with a combination of estramustine, vinblastine, mitozantrone, and hydrocortisone[7]. To date these are small studies requiring further investigation to establish the true role of strontium in combination with chemotherapy.

The second approach has evaluated high-dose rhenium using peripheral blood stem cell support in an attempt to deliver ablative doses to the bone metastasis[8]. Early studies suggest this is a feasible technique with satisfactory bone marrow recovery and efficacy data are awaited.

6.2.3 Prophylactic

Radioisotopes, in particular strontium, have been evaluated as a means of slowing and preventing symptoms arising from asymptomatic bone metastasis. The Trans Canada study was a large randomized phase III trial in which patients with hormone resistant prostate cancer receiving local radiotherapy for a painful bone metastasis in the setting of other asymptomatic multiple metastasis were randomized to receive additional strontium or placebo[4]. Significantly fewer new symptomatic bone metastasis were seen in the strontium group and a reduced need for further treatment was found. A similar reduction in new symptomatic sites has been found in both prospective[9] and retrospective case–control studies[10] in patients with hormone refractory prostate cancer comparing strontium and palliative local radiotherapy. While no difference in disease free or overall survival is noted in these studies there does appear to be a preventive effect from using intravenous strontium in asymptomatic metastasis, the magnitude of which is modest. This is not a common indication for its use.

Table 6.2 Doses of isotopes in current clinical use for metastatic bone pain

Strontium chloride	^{89}Sr	150 MBq
Samarium-EDTMP	^{153}Sm	37 MBq/kg (1 mCi/kg)
Rhenium HEDP	^{186}Re	1295 MBq
Rhenium HEDP	^{189}Re	3.3–4.4 GBq

6.3 **Doses**

Standard doses used in clinical practice are based on maximum tolerated doses defined by bone marrow toxicity. These are shown in Table 6.2.

6.4 **Precautions and toxicity**

The radioisotopes in common clinical use are strontium and samarium. Rhenium is also available in many European countries and the USA. As with any radioisotope administration this should be undertaken with appropriate supervision by medical physics personnel adhering to the pertinent radiation protection regulations. These are described fully in Chapter 9. Both isotopes are given intravenously as a bolus injection and precautions similar to those used for the administration of chemotherapy should be adopted ensuring a safe intravenous cannula is placed into a large peripheral vein with patency checked by saline flush or a slow running infusion of saline. The bolus injection should be washed through the cannula with further saline.

Absolute contraindications are patients with spinal cord compression, those who are pregnant, and those who wish to continue breast feeding.

The isotopes are predominantly beta emitters and therefore adequate protection for the administrating physician is provided by a lead shielded syringe.

Clinical toxicity is unusual with these agents, which are generally very well tolerated. No immediate side-effects are usually seen after the intravenous administration. Strontium being a pure beta emitter has no restricting radiation protection issue and patients can be treated as an outpatient and allowed home immediately including those who have to travelled on public transport. The physical half-life of ^{89}Sr is 50.5 days and it is cleared from the plasma with a mean elimination half-life of 47 hours. This is predominantly renal clearance, the major radiation hazard therefore being excreted isotope in the urine. Small amounts are also excreted into the gut and in sweat. Renal tubular reabsorption occurs under the control of parathyroid hormone, which accounts for the individual variation in renal clearance. The decay product of strontium, yttrium, is also excreted in urine. The biological half-life in normal bone is about 14 days, compared with over 50 days in osteoblastic metastases.

Samarium in contrast has a much shorter half-life of 46.3 days emitting predominantly beta energy but also low-energy 103 KeV gamma photons. Higher radiation doses of samarium are given but it is cleared rapidly with a plasma elimination half-life achieving 85% clearance within 30 minutes. Only 1% of the dose remains in plasma 1 hour after administration. Mean skeletal uptake has been estimated to reflect 65% ± 15.5% of the administered dose and distribution in the skeleton can be accurately predicted from ^{99M}Tc MDP uptake on a diagnostic isotope bone scan as shown in Fig. 6.1. As for strontium the principal route of excretion is urinary and its rapid elimination results in completion of urinary excretion within 6 hours. Prehydration with 500 ml of fluid is recommended and some studies have used more rigorous pre- and posthydration schedules for up to 6 hours after administration. The higher dose and gamma emission from samarium does introduce additional radiation protection considerations and the standard recommendation is for the patient to be monitored within the hospital environment for 6 hours after administration with supervised disposal of their urine.

The dependence of both strontium and samarium on renal excretion for plasma elimination means that adequate renal function is a critical requirement for the safe administration of these isotopes. Patients with impaired renal function should not receive this treatment.

Rhenium is used in two isotope forms; ^{186}Re has a half-life of 89 hours with a biological half-life in bone metastases of up to 59 hours in osteoblastic metastases from prostate cancer. ^{188}Re has a short physical half-life of only 16.9 hours. It is produced in a rhenium generator by decay from Tungsten ^{188}W, thus providing an efficient and cost-effective source of radioisotope, independent of nuclear reactor capacity and suitable for use in relatively under developed healthcare scenarios once the investment in the generator has been made.

6.5 Clinical toxicity

6.5.1 Bone pain flare

Exacerbation of bone pain is a recognized phenomenon with both isotopes. It is reported after strontium in about 15% of patients developing in the first 5 days after administration with a duration of about 4 days. One study has suggested this may be associated with a better subsequent response in terms of pain relief[11]. Flare after samarium is reported in 12–20% of patients with a similar time profile[3] and in up to 50% of patients after rhenium[2]. There are no recognized predictive factors for those patients who will develop pain flare and management relies on warning patients of the possibility and ensuring they have access to adequate supplementary analgesia for that short period.

6.5.2 Bone marrow depression

Both isotopes deliver radiation doses to the bone marrow. There is a wide variation of absorbed dose from the isotope. Strontium uptake into bone metastasis is two to 25 times greater than into normal bone and retention in bone metastasis at 100 days has been estimated between 0.7% and 2.9% of an administered dose. The absorbed dose varies widely, one estimate for vertebral dose ranging from 6 cGy/MBq to 610 cGy/MBq with a ratio of tumour dose to marrow dose of 1–10. The retention in metastasis is inversely proportional to the extent of metastasis and this partly defines the wide variation of absorbed dose[12].

Similarly the total skeletal dose of samarium varies widely, the mean skeletal uptake representing 65.5% of the administered dose with a ratio of bone marrow to bone metastasis doses of 1:5. The range of uptake may vary from 15% to 95% with a tumour/normal bone ratio of 5:1[13].

Clinical bone marrow depression is usually only moderate and rarely results in major sequelae. Transient falls in both peripheral white cell count and platelets are to be expected in 80% of patients receiving standard doses of strontium and a similar proportion of patients receiving samarium. Typically this will be a fall to about 50% of the pretreatment value with the nadir being reached at 4 weeks after administration and recovery by 8 weeks. Provided patients have normal renal function at the outset more serious reductions in platelet count causing bleeding or neutropenia causing sepsis are not expected. Transient falls in haemoglobin are also seen. About 10% of patients may develop grade III or IV haemoglobin toxicity, requiring blood transfusion.

Bone marrow problems are most likely in patients who have borderline renal function and those with pre-existing compromise to bone marrow function often due to preceding extensive external beam radiotherapy or chemotherapy. Increased toxicity has been reported in patients with subclinical disseminated intravascular coagulation, which is relatively common in patients with prostate cancer[14].

There is a theoretical risk of leukaemia induction; there are two cases reported after administration of strontium against a background of pretreatment with both chemotherapy and external beam radiotherapy[15]. The majority of patients are treated in the final stages of their malignancy and this is therefore not a significant risk; however, it may be a factor to be considered where earlier use of radioisotope therapy is recommended.

Mild flushing has been reported at the time of injection of strontium, which is transient and self-limiting. Other significant toxicities are not recognized.

6.6 Clinical efficacy

6.6.1 Strontium

The evaluation of strontium has been predominantly in patients with metastatic prostate cancer with hormone resistant disease and metastatic bone pain. In a prospective randomized double-blind crossover study using stable ^{88}Sr as the control group significantly better pain control and reduced analgesic intake was found after both the initial treatment period and at the end of the crossover period in the group receiving active ^{89}Sr[16]. Two large studies have compared ^{89}Sr with external beam radiotherapy. The first of these[9] stratified patients into those requiring local treatment and those requiring hemibody external beam radiotherapy and compared both modalities against strontium. No statistically significant differences in pain relief or analgesic use were found between the four groups. The second study[10] randomized patients to receive either ^{89}Sr or local radiotherapy and again no significant difference in rates of pain relief or time to progression were found. This study did, however, report an improvement in median survival in patients receiving external radiotherapy compared with strontium with a 1-year survival of 45% compared with 34%. No such effect was seen in the other study and no clear explanation has emerged for this survival difference. No significant differences in toxicity, including blood product requirements were seen between strontium and local radiotherapy in either study, although in the study in which hemibody radiotherapy was included the bone marrow toxicity in that group was significantly greater.

The average time to onset of pain relief is 10–14 days with a range of 4–28 days and response duration may be up to 15 months. This implies that the utility of strontium for patients with a predicted life expectancy of less than 2–3 months is low and it should only be considered after careful consideration and patient selection in this setting. Greatest clinical effect is seen in patients with good performance status, limited skeletal involvement, haemoglobin >10 g/dl and prostate-specific antigen levels <100 μg/l[17].

Two studies have looked at ^{89}Sr as an adjuvant to radiotherapy. The first of these was the Trans Canada study in which 126 patients were randomized after receiving local radiotherapy for bone pain to receive adjuvant ^{89}Sr or placebo[4]. The dose delivered in this study was higher than the standard dose, 400 MBq. A higher incidence of pain relief was obtained in the strontium group (40% at 3 months compared with 23% in the placebo group) and fewer new sites of pain developed in those patients who receive strontium. The second study reported from Norway[18] randomized only 95 patients before closing due to poor accrual. While no difference in pain relief scores was found the study was underpowered to reach a definitive conclusion.

A limited number of studies have looked at other primary sites, particularly breast cancer with a small number of patients having lung cancer and other primary sites included. These suggest the response rates and patterns of response are similar in those cancers as would be expected as the pathophysiology of bone metastasis is similar independent of the primary site. The largest of these[19] comprising 229 patients reported response rates of 69% in prostate cancer, 64% in breast cancer, and 50% in other cancers.

6.6.2 Samarium

The studies in samarium have been less tumour site specific but have again focused primarily on patients with primary tumours of prostate and breast. A large prospective randomized double blind trial of samarium EDTMP comparing the active form [^{153}Sm] with an inactive form [^{152}Sm] included 152 patients with hormone refractory prostate cancer[20]. Statistically significant reductions in pain scale and opioid use were seen within the first 4 weeks after administration associated with transient falls in blood count with no grade IV toxicity. The incidence of pain flare in this study was 6%. A similar study, which included prostate, breast, and other cancers, compared two doses of samarium with placebo and reported an overall response rate of 65% with 31% of patients achieving complete response at 4 weeks after receiving the higher dose of 1 mCi/kg, a statistically significant improvement over the placebo complete response of 14%[21]. Similar results have been reported from smaller phase II trials and a phase III dose finding trial[22]. The overall response rate for a dose of 1 mCi/kg (37 MBq/kg) ranging from 70 to 83% and including patients with prostate, breast, and other primary sites.

Overall, the pattern of response seen with samarium is similar to that with strontium. It has been proposed a more rapid onset of pain relief may be a feature of samarium related to the higher dose rate but simple comparison of published response rates in studies of samarium and those with strontium suggests there is no major difference.

6.6.3 Rhenium

There are two active isotopes of rhenium, ^{186}Re and ^{188}Re. The isotope most commonly evaluated in clinical use has been ^{186}Re complexed with II-hydroethylidene disphosphonate (Re HEDP). Both rhenium isotopes produce low-energy gamma irradiation and can be imaged. An example is shown in Fig. 6.2. One double-blind randomized phase III trial has confirmed the efficacy of rhenium over placebo in patients with metastatic prostate cancer[23] and a smaller crossover study confirmed greater pain relief with rhenium [186]Re HEDP than placebo[24]. Smaller phase II studies suggest overall pain responses of between 38 and 82% with a similar onset in duration to that seen with strontium and similar profile of pain flare and side-effects[1].

The main application of [188]Re to date has been in a small number of dose finding and phase II studies in which overall the pattern of response appears similar to that of the other radiopharmaceuticals used for metastatic bone pain but there is insufficient evidence at present to consider it for routine clinical use.

6.6.4 Tin ([117]Sn)

[117]Sn produces very short-range beta particles penetrating <1 mm; this may have potential benefit in producing less bone marrow suppression. Early data suggest that it has efficacy in bone metastases but there are no phase III data yet available to confirm this against placebo or control.

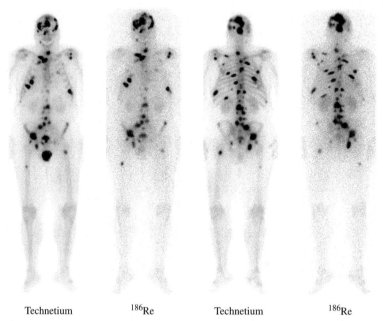

Technetium   [186]Re   Technetium   [186]Re

Fig. 6.2 Rhenium uptake in bone metastases demonstrated on gamma camera pictures alongside diagnostic technetium images (courtesy of Dr C. Hoefnagel, the Netherlands Cancer Institute).

6.6.5 **Radium (^{223}Ra)**

^{223}Ra is unique among the radioisotopes used for bone metastases in that its therapeutic radiation is in the form of alpha particles. These have two potential advantages; the first is that of short range, of the order of 100 nm, again potentially minimizing bone marrow toxicity. The second lies in the higher linear energy transfer of alpha compared with beta and gamma radiation, which means that it has greater relative biological effectiveness dose for dose. Early phase I work with this isotope suggests it is effective and safe in humans and further trials are currently under way.

6.7 **Retreatment**

In selected patients retreatment is both feasible and effective. Provided patients continue to fulfil the criteria for safe radioisotope administration and there has been no deterioration in renal function, the only requirement is that a sufficient interval has been allowed for bone marrow recovery; typically retreatment after 3 months is entirely safe and effective.

6.8 **Comparison between radioisotopes**

Two studies have compared the use of strontium and rhenium. Neither of these is randomized and their validity is therefore limited; one included 527 treatments with strontium and 83 with rhenium[25], the second 29 with strontium and 31 with rhenium[26]. No difference in efficacy or toxicity was demonstrated, however, although there was a suggestion that strontium results in a slightly longer duration of response than rhenium. A third non-randomized study reported the use of ^{186}Re in 13 patients, ^{188}Re in 15 patients and strontium in 16 patients[27]. Response rates of 77–81% were seen with similar degrees of platelet reduction after therapy.

6.9 **Combination therapy with chemotherapy**

Radioisotope therapy is of limited efficacy in terms of tumour cell kill when used alone and it has therefore been proposed that the use of combination therapy with chemotherapy may be advantageous. Two small phase II studies have been published with strontium combined with either doxorubicin or cisplatin in prostatic cancer. The first of these reported on 103 patients treated with induction chemotherapy from whom 72 were responders or had stable disease after two cycles. These patients were randomized to receive doxorubicin weekly for 6 weeks alone or with a single administration of strontium. Survival in the combined therapy group was 27.7 months compared with 16.8 months in the doxorubicin alone group[5]. The second randomized

70 patients with hormone resistant prostate cancer to receive either strontium alone or strontium with cisplatin 50 mg/m². Survival in the combined group was 9 months compared with 6 months in the strontium alone group[6]. These observations have stimulated a number of phase III trials currently underway to explore this approach.

6.9.1 **High-dose radioisotope therapy**

The use of marrow ablative doses of chemotherapy using peripheral blood stem cell support is well established. Analogous to this high-dose radioisotope therapy is currently being explored as a potential means of targeting micrometastases in bone using either samarium or rhenium[8].

6.9.2 **Osteosarcoma**

One additional indication for bone seeking radioisotope therapy is in the treatment of osteosarcoma, particularly recurrent and metastatic disease. A characteristic of osteosarcoma is osteoblastic activity with the formation of osteoid, a feature that will also enable concentration of these isotopes at sites of active tumour. Thus the paradoxical observation of strontium or samarium EDTMP in lung metastases has been described with effective palliation achieved in their use for metastatic disease no longer suitable for chemotherapy[28]. The role of radioisotope therapy in the radical treatment programmes for osteoblastoma has yet to be evaluated.

6.10 **Alternative treatments and cost effectiveness**

Strontium, samarium, and rhenium are effective agents for the treatment of metastatic bone pain. The overall picture suggests response rates similar to that seen with external beam radiotherapy with 70–80% of patients reporting pain relief using various parameters and up to 30% complete pain relief, albeit using different definitions in different studies. There may be a more rapid onset of pain relief with samarium and rhenium when overall pain relief is seen within the first few weeks after administration and maintained for several months. Equally rapid responses may be seen with wide field radiotherapy, 25% of patients reporting response in the first 24 hours after treatment[28].

There is limited experience with repeated isotope administration and the general recommendation is to defer further administration until bone marrow recovery has been seen and typically this will be 6–12 weeks after the first administration. This then clearly selects out a group of patients with a particularly good prognosis who will still have good performance status

3 months on from their first treatment for scattered metastatic bone pain in whom repeated administration may be of value.

It has been suggested that because of their higher dose rate and shorter beta range samarium and rhenium should be considered for patients with severe pain and a heavy metastatic burden with reduced marrow reserve, while strontium is more suitable for earlier treatment in patients with a lesser metastatic load and good bone marrow reserve. In practice this choice is likely to be influenced as much by cost, isotope availability, and radioprotection issues.

Similar results are obtained with external beam radiotherapy and with radionuclide therapy. There is no evidence to suggest that one modality is more effective than the other provided external beam radiotherapy is given to an appropriate volume, and where there are several sites of pain wide field or hemibody treatment is considered. Hemibody radiotherapy, however, is associated with greater gastrointestinal toxicity in contrast to that seen after standard doses of radioisotope and local external beam radiotherapy. Radioisotope treatment, particularly using strontium, which does not require any additional radioprotection restriction, is clearly easier for the patient who attends for a single outpatient intravenous injection compared with the more complex procedure of external beam radiotherapy planning and administration; this advantage is even greater where multifraction schedules for metastatic bone pain are still in use.

Radioisotopes are more expensive to deliver as a single dose than a single dose of external beam radiotherapy. A cost–benefit analysis of the Trans Canada study in which the reduction in requirements for further treatment was offset against the addition of strontium revealed that strontium in that setting could be cost-effective[4]. For the patient with several sites of metastatic bone pain for whom the choice of effective treatment is a single exposure of hemibody radiotherapy compared with a single injection of a radioisotope, the external beam treatment is undoubtedly less costly at the point of treatment delivery although associated with greater toxicity. A cost–benefit study has also been undertaken using data from the Dutch trial of strontium[29] and concluded that strontium was 25% more expensive than external beam radiotherapy as delivered in the Dutch healthcare system.

The bisphosphonate drugs may also be considered as an alternative to radioisotopes in the setting of multisite metastatic bone pain. Their relative efficacy for the relief of bone pain has not been tested and published reports suggest that response rates are in general under 50%[30]. They undoubtedly have a prophylactic effect reducing the progression of bone metastasis where they are established or in high-risk patients by other criteria. In this setting, however, their regular use for 1 or 2 years is a substantial cost to the health economy against which the use of a single radioisotope injection may be seen as highly cost-effective. Their major advantage lies in their ease of administration requiring no medical physics support or supervised administration, and carrying no radioprotection concerns. For this reason they are often given prior to the consideration of radioisotopes or alongside them but this practice cannot be recommended on the basis of the published data at present.

There are patients who are less likely to benefit from radioisotopes and others in whom the cost and the radiation exposure cannot be justified. These will include those with poor performance status (WHO grade II or worse), advanced soft tissue metastatic disease, those with pathological fracture or spinal cord compression and where the pain has a substantial mechanical component or is due to underlying degenerative or osteoporotic disease. However, for those with good performance status, a predicted survival of >2 months, limited uncomplicated bone metastases and controlled or absent soft tissue disease in whom scattered metastatic bone pain is the predominant symptom, intravenous radioisotopes will make a substantial contribution to their management.

References

1. Bauman G, Charette M, Reid R, Sathya J (2005). Radiopharmaceuticals for the palliation of painful bone metastases—a systematic review. *Radiotherapy and Oncology* **75**: 258–70.

2. Lewington VJ (2005). Bone-seeking radionuclides for therapy. *Journal of Nuclear Medicine* **46**: 38–47S.

3. Finlay IG, Mason MD, Shelley M (2005). Radioisotopes for the palliation of metastatic bone cancer: a systematic review. *Lancet Oncology* **6**: 392–400.

4. Porter AT, McEwan AJ (1993). Strontium-89 as an adjuvant to external beam radiation improves pain relief and delays disease progression in advanced prostate cancer: results of a randomized controlled trial. *Seminars in Oncology* **20**: 38–43.

5. Tu SM, Millikan RE, Mengistu B *et al.* (2001). Bone-targeted therapy for advanced androgen-independent carcinoma of the prostate: a randomised phase II trial. *Lancet* **357**: 336–41.

6. Sciuto R, Festa A, Rea S, *et al.* (2002). Effects of low-dose cisplatin on 89Sr therapy for painful bone metastases from prostate cancer: a randomized clinical trial. *Journal of Nuclear Medicine* **43**: 79–86.

7. Akerley W, Butera J, Wehbe T *et al.* (2002). A multiinstitutional, concurrent chemoradiation trial of strontium-89, estramustine, and vinblastine for hormone refractory prostate carcinoma involving bone. *Cancer* **94**: 1654–60.

8. O'Sullivan JM, McCreday VR, Flux G, *et al.* (2002). High activity rhenium 186 HEDP with autologous peripheral stem cell rescue: a phase I study in progressive hormone refractory prostate cancer metastatic to bone. *Br J Cancer* **86**: 1715–20.

9. Quilty PM, Kirk D, Bolger JJ, *et al.* (1994). A comparison of the palliative effects of strontium-89 and external beam radiotherapy in metastatic prostate cancer. *Radiotherapy and Oncology* **31**: 33–40.

10. Dearnaley DP, Bayly RJ, A'Hern RP, *et al.* (1992). Palliation of bone metastases in prostate cancer. Hemibody irradiation or strontium-89? *Clinical Oncology* **4**: 101–7.

11. Laing AH, Ackery DM, Bayly RJ *et al.* (1991). Strontium-89 chloride for pain palliation in prostatic skeletal malignancy. *British Journal of Radiology* **64**: 816–22.

12. Hoskin PJ (1994). Strontium. In: Dollery C (ed.), *Drugs and Therapeutics Supplement I*, pp. 223–6. Edinburgh: Churchill Livingstone.

13. Quadramet monograph, Cis Bio International (1998).

14. Pazkowski AL, Hewitt DJ, Taylor A Jr *et al.* (1999). Disseminated intravascular coagulation in a patient treated with strontium-89 for metastatic carcinoma of the prostate. *Clinical Nuclear Medicine* **24**: 852–4.

15. Kossman SE, Weiss MA (2000). Acute myelogenous leukaemia after exposure to strontium 89 for the treatment of adenocarcinoma of the prostate. *Cancer* **88**: 620–4.

16. Lewington VJ, McEwan AJ, Ackery DM, *et al.* (1991). A prospective, randomised double-blind crossover study to examine the efficacy of strontium-89 in pain palliation in patients with advanced prostate cancer metastatic to bone. *European Journal of Cancer* **27**: 954–8.

17. Windsor PM (2001). Predictors of response to strontium-89 (Metastron®) in skeletal metastases from prostate cancer: report of a single centre's 10-year experience. *Clinical Oncology* **13**: 219–27.

18. Smeland S, Erikstein B, Aas M, *et al.* (2003). Role of strontium-89 as adjuvant to palliative external beam radiotherapy is questionable: results of a double-blind randomized study. *International Journal of Radiation Oncology, Biology, Physics* **56**: 1397–404.

19. Blitzer PH, Dosoretz DE, Floody PA, *et al.* (1995). Strontium-89 chloride in the palliation of bone pain from metastatic cancer. *Proceedings of the American Society of Clinical Oncology* **14**: 511 (Abstr. 1678).

20. Sartor O, Reid RH, Hoskin PJ, *et al.* (2004). Samarium-153-Lexidronam complex for treatment of painful bone metastases in hormone-refractory prostate cancer. *Urology* **63**: 940–5.

21. Serafini AN, Houston SJ, Resche I, *et al.* (1998). Palliation of pain associated with metastatic bone cancer using samarium-153 lexidronam: a double-blind placebo-controlled clinical trial. *Journal of Clinical Oncology* **16**: 1574–81.

22. Olea E, Riccabona G, Tian J, *et al.* (2000). Efficacy and toxicity of 153Sm EDTMP in the palliative treatment of painful skeleton metastases: results of an IAEA international multicenter study. *Journal of Nuclear Medicine* **51**: 146 (Abstr.).

23. Han SH, de Klerk JMH, Tan S, *et al.* (2002). The placorhen study: a double-blind, placebo-controlled, randomized radionuclide study with 186Re-etidronate in hormone-resistant prostate cancer patients with painful bone metastases. *Journal of Nuclear Medicine* **43**: 1150–6.

24. Maxon III RH, Schroder LE, Hertzberg VS, *et al.* (1991). Rhenium-186(Sn)HEDP for treatment of painful osseous metastases: results of a double-blind crossover comparison with placebo. *Journal of Nuclear Medicine* **32**: 1877–81.

25. Dafermou A, Colamussi P, Giganti M, *et al.* (2001). A multicentre observational study of radionuclide therapy in patients with painful bone metastases of prostate cancer. *Eur Journal of Nuclear Medicine* **28**: 788–98.

26. van der Poel HG, Antonini N, Hoefnagel CA *et al.* (2006). Serum hemoglobin levels predict resource to strontium-89 and rhenium-186-HEDP radionuclide treatment for painful osseous metastases in prostate cancer. *Urol. Int.* **77**: 50–56.

27. Liepe K, Franke WG, Kropp J, Koch R, Runge R, Hliscs R (2000). Comparison of rhenium-188, rhenium-186-HEDP and strontium-89 in palliation of painful bone metastases. *Nuklearmedizin* **39**(6): 146–51.

28. Hoskin PJ, Ford HT, Harmer CL (1989). Hemibody irradiation for metastatic bone pain in two histologically distinct groups of patients. *Clinical Oncology* **1**; 67–9.

29. Oosterhof GON, Roberts JT, De Reijke T, *et al.* (2003). Strontium[89] chloride versus palliative local field radiotherapy in patients with hormonal escaped prostate cancer: a phase III study of the European organisation for research and treatment of cancer genitourinary group. *European Urology* **44**: 519–26.

30. Hoskin PJ (2003). Radiotherapy and bisphosphonates in the management of bone metastases. *Cancer Treatment Reviews* **29**: 321–7.

Chapter 7

Radioimmunotherapy for lymphoma

Tim Illidge, Yong Du

7.1 Background to use

7.1.1 Non-Hodgkin lymphoma

Non-Hodgkin lymphoma (NHL) represents a group of lymphoid malignancies that traverse a broad clinical spectrum ranging from indolent disease with a long natural history such as low-grade follicular lymphoma to very aggressive 'high grade' but potentially curable diseases such as Burkitt's lymphoma[1]. NHL is largely a disease of older adults, with a peak incidence in individuals greater than 60 years of age. It is the fifth and sixth most common malignancy in females and males, respectively, and the NHL are responsible for 4% of all cancers and 4% of cancer deaths seen in the US[2]. The incidence of NHL has been continuously on the rise over the past 25 years and the reasons for this remain largely unknown. Data collected from the Survival, Epidemiology, and End Results (SEER) project demonstrated a twofold rise in incidence (8/100 000 to 16/100 000) between 1973 and 1995. A majority of 85% of NHL are B lymphocyte origin while T lymphocytes, natural killer cells or unknown cell type origins form the rest 15%[3,4]. Although observational data have demonstrated an association between NHL and several toxic exposures, immune defects, or infectious diseases; however the cause of NHL in most individuals is unknown.

The recognition and description of such heterogeneous lymphoma types has evolved over many years. Currently, the 'World Health Organization Classification Scheme for Non-Hodgkin's Lymphoma'[5,6] is widely accepted and is a largely successful attempt to integrate clinical and new pathological information into one classification. A much simplified version is shown in Table 7.1.

Despite the sensitivity of most lymphomas to initial therapy with chemotherapy or radiotherapy, the majority of patients with advanced NHL eventually relapse and die of their disease[1]. Furthermore, patients with

Table 7.1 Word Health Organization Classification Scheme of the more common non-Hodgkin's lymphoma

B-cell neoplasms	Frequency (%)
Mature B-cell neoplasms	
B-cell chronic lymphocytic leukaemia/small lymphocytic lymphoma	7%
Lymphoplasmacytic lymphoma	1.5%
Extranodal marginal zone B-cell lymphoma of MALT type	10%
Follicular lymphoma	25%
Mantle-cell lymphoma	5–7%
Diffuse large B-cell lymphoma	31%
Burkitt's lymphoma	2%
Other rarer lymphomas	
T-cell and NK-cell neoplasms	15%

HTLV-1, human T-cell leukaemia virus 1; MALT, mucosa-associated lymphoid tissue; NK, natural killer.

advanced low-grade lymphomas remain incurable and their survival has not altered since the early 1960s. The introduction of monoclonal antibody (mAb) based therapy and more recently radioimmunotherapy (RIT) has provided fresh hope for NHL patients that their prognosis can be improved.

7.1.2 Antibody-targeted therapy in non-Hodgkin lymphoma

Following the advent of mAb technology in the 1970s[7], there was a great expectation that mAb would provide effective targeted therapy for cancer. Over the past three decades, there has been intense therapeutic evaluation of a wide spectrum of mAb recognizing different tumour-specific or tumour-associated antigens. Finally in 1997, rituximab, a mAb directed against the CD20 antigen on the surface of B cells was approved by the US Food and Drug Administration (US FDA) for the treatment of cancer and thus provided a very significant milestone in the history of targeted therapy. Rituximab has subsequently been successfully used in a wide variety of B-cell malignancies[8]. The single agent response rates of rituximab, however, remains rather modest, with overall response rates in the order of about 50% and complete response (CR) rates usually in single figures for previously treated patients with follicular lymphoma[9,10]. Therefore to increase response rates mAb are increasingly being given with chemotherapy or radiotherapy.

RIT is a conceptually appealing approach for cancer treatment whereby the conjugation of radioisotope to mAb enables the delivery of targeted radiotherapy in addition to the specific cytotoxic effects of the mAb. Over the last few years RIT has been shown to demonstrate vastly superior clinical responses to unlabelled anti-CD20 mAb[11,12]. A wide variety of different mAb, delivery schedules, radioisotopes, and doses of radioactivity have been used in RIT and have resulted in impressive durable partial responses (PRs) and CRs in the treatment of NHL[11,13,14]. It now seems highly likely that RIT will play a significant part in the treatment of some NHL following the US FDA approval of two RIT drugs namely ^{90}Y-ibritumomab tiuxetan and ^{131}I-tositumomab. This chapter will thus focus on the clinical indications for these two radioimmunoconjugates, the efficacy data that led to approval, the differences in dosimetry and delivery of the two drugs and their side-effect profiles.

7.1.3 The principles of radioimmunotherapy

RIT has come to refer to the therapeutic administration of radionuclides chemically conjugated to mAb or mAb-derived constructs. mAb can be generated to recognize and bind to either tumour-specific antigens or antigens that are highly expressed on tumour cells. mAb were initially regarded simply as direct carriers for the radionuclide that delivers systemically targeted radiation to areas of disease with relative sparing of normal tissue. It is, however, becoming clearer that the mAb effector mechanisms may also play an important additional role in killing lymphoma cells. The nature of RIT determines that its efficacy depends on a number of factors, including properties of the targeted antigen (specificity, density, availability, shedding, and heterogeneity of expression), the tumour (vascularity, blood flow, and permeability), the mAb (specificity, immunoreactivity, stability, and affinity), and the properties of chosen radionuclides (emission characteristics, half-life and availability)[15].

Tumour-specific antigens would be the ideal targets, but that degree of specificity is unusual and in practice tumour-associated antigens, expressed abundantly on tumour cells as well as some normal tissues represent the majority of potential targets. As most NHL are of B-cell origin the pan-B-cell antigens such as human leukocyte antigen DR (HLA-DR), CD19, CD20, CD22, CD37, and CD52 have been extensively evaluated as targets for RIT[16–24]. Among them, CD20 has many of the characteristics thought to be important for an ideal target (Table 7.2)[25], which does not internalize or shed from the cell surface and initiates signal transduction that triggers apoptosis through a caspase-dependent pathway[26,27]. CD20 is highly expressed on the majority of B-cell lymphomas but not expressed on stem cells or plasma cells so that after treatment the B-cell pool is replenished. Currently, anti-CD20

Table 7.2 The characteristics of an ideal target antigen

Tumour cell specific
Highly expressed on tumour cells
No tendency to mutation
Not secreted or shed
Not rapidly modulated on antibody binding
Critical for target cell survival
Not expressed on critical or non renewable host cells

mAb-directed approaches dominate clinical RIT of NHL, although other antigens such as the CD22 are being actively investigated[28,29].

7.2 Clinical indications

90Y-ibritumomab tiuxetan (Zevalin®) was the first of this class of drugs to be licensed by the US FDA and is currently the only radioimmunoconjugate to be licensed within the EU. However, both 90Y-ibritumomab tiuxetan and 131I-tositumomab (Bexxar®) are approved for the treatment of adult patients with relapsed CD20-positive follicular or transformed B-cell NHL within the USA. The licence for 90Y-ibritumomab tiuxetan within the EU is restricted to relapsed follicular lymphoma, which is refractory to or relapsed after rituximab. The characteristics of both 90Y-ibritumomab tiuxetan and 131I-tositumomab are shown in Table 7.3 and the most noticeable difference is regarding the 4–5 days in patient stay within the EU required for 131I-tositumomab, which contrasts to a single outpatient is required for the delivery of 90Y Ibirtumomab.

Patients with an increased likelihood of developing haematological toxicity or patients with impaired bone marrow reserve as defined by the following criteria should be excluded from treatment RIT with 131I-tositumomab or 90Y-ibritumomab. The current exclusions based on bone marrow biopsy are listed below.

♦ presence of >25% infiltration of lymphoma cells within the bone marrow

♦ hypocellular bone marrow (<15% cellularity)

♦ marked reduction of bone marrow precursors.

Impaired bone marrow reserves as indicated by:

♦ prior myeloablative therapies with allogeneic bone marrow (ABM) or peripheral blood stem cell (PBSC) transplantation

♦ platelet count <100 000 cells/mm^3

♦ ANC (neutrophil count (absolute)) <1500 cells/mm^3

Table 7.3 Characteristics of ^{131}I-tositumomab (Bexxar^{TM}) and ^{90}Y-ibritumomab tiuxetan (Zevalin^{TM})

	^{131}I-tositumomab	^{90}Y-ibritumomab tiuxetan
US Trade name	Bexxar	Zevalin
Monoclonal antibody	Tositumomab (anti-B1)—murine	Ibritumomab (2B8)—murine
Chelation	Simple	More complex
Isotope	^{131}I	^{90}Y
Isotope emissions	γ and β	β only
β energy	0.606 MeV	2.293 MeV
β particle path length	0.8 mm	5.3 mm
Isotope half-life	8 days	2.6 days
γ energy,	0.364 MeV	None
Radiation protection measures	4–6-day inpatient stay in shielded room	Outpatient
Isotope excretion	Renal (variable)	Limited
Normal tissue uptake	Thyroid (blocked with potassium iodate)	Bone
Pre-dose (unlabelled antibody)	Tositumomab (450 mg/patient)	Rituximab (250 mg/m^2) × 2
Dose	75 cGy whole body dose Dosimetric dose obligatory	0.4 mCi/kg Dosimetric dose not required Dose reduction for thrombocytopenia

♦ patients with a platelet count between 100 000 and 150 000/µl should be given a dose reduction of ^{90}Y-ibritumomab to 0.3 mCi/kg (11.1 MBq/kg) and 65 cGy whole body dose for ^{131}I-tositumomab.

A further exclusion is impaired renal function defined by:

♦ serum creatinine >1.5 × the upper limit of normal.

All patients require a bone marrow trephine examination within 4–6 weeks prior to treatment with RIT. Patients should be excluded if pregnant or breast feeding, or if known to have hypersensitivity to mouse antibodies or chelating agents like tiuxetan or serum human antimurine antibody (HAMA). Patients with known active infection with the human immunodeficiency virus, or lymphoma of the central nervous system should also be excluded, as there are currently no data to confirm the safety of this approach in these groups of patients. Patients who progressed within 1 year of radiation in a field that had been previously been irradiated or who were receiving other anticancer drugs or biologics were not eligible. It is recommended that prior chemotherapy must have been discontinued ≥4 weeks (6 weeks for nitrosourea compounds) before RIT.

Despite initial concerns, preliminary data suggest that patients after prior bone marrow transplant or stem cell support can be safely treated as long as a significant dose reduction is made. For ^{90}Y-ibritumomab tiuxetan regimen the published data at present suggest a dose of 0.2 mCi/kg and for ^{131}I-tositumomab about 65 cGy whole body dose to be feasible[30,31]. It should be emphasized that the delivery of either RIT drug postautologous stem cell transplantation is outside of the current licensed indication.

7.3 **Typical doses**

7.3.1 **Radioisotopes used in radioimmunotherapy**

The optimal radionuclide delivers the maximal dose of ionizing radiation to tumour sites while minimizing the radiation dose to normal tissue and to medical personnel. The physical characteristics considered important for a radionuclide in RIT include half-life, type of radioactive emissions (α, β, or γ), and ionization path length. Particle energy and mean path length in tissue are important determinants of therapeutic efficacy. The emission profile of radionuclide not only determines its suitability for therapy, but also the toxicological profile.

Animal studies have consistently indicated that the major dose-limiting organ for RIT is the bone marrow[32]. With the advent of bone marrow and peripheral blood stem cell transplantation, the upper limit of the amount of tolerable radiation dose is likely to increase[28].

The most frequently used radionuclides and their physical characteristics are listed in Table 7.4.

In practice, the choice of the optimal isotope for RIT remains controversial, with proponents advocating the relative merits of ^{131}I, ^{90}Y, ^{186}Re, ^{67}Cu, and α emitters such as ^{211}At[28]. Comparative studies are difficult to conduct and scientifically sound randomized human trials have not been performed.

The majority of clinical trials to date have used either ^{131}I or ^{90}Y because of their favourable emission characteristics, availability, and well documented radiochemistry that permit reliable and stable attachment to mAb. ^{131}I has the advantage of a long history of successful use in the management of

Table 7.4 Physical characteristics of radioisotopes used in RIT

Radioisotope	Half-life	Emission		Path length
131I	8.1 days	β	0.6 MeV*	0.8 mm
		γ (81%)	0.37 MeV	
90Y	2.5 days	β	2.3 MeV	5.3 mm
		γ	nil	
186Re	3.7 days	β	1.1 MeV	1.8 mm
		γ (9%)	0.14 MeV	
125I	60.1 days	Electron capture	7.45 MeV	0.001 mm
		γ	0.027 MeV	
67Cu	2.5 days	β	0.4-0.6 MeV	0.6 mm
		γ	0.185 MeV	
211At	7 hours	α	6.8 MeV	0.065 mm
		Electron capture	7.45 MeV	
213Bi	1 hour	α	7.8 MeV	0.07 mm
		γ	0.72 MeV	

*Million Electron Volts

thyroid cancer and a well documented safety profile. It is readily available, inexpensive, easily conjugated, and emits both β particles with a path length of 0.8 mm and penetrating γ emissions. The γ emissions enable uncomplicated imaging using gamma camera for dosimetry purposes but result in a significant non-targeted normal tissue radiation dose, as well as radiation protection issues for visitors and medical/nursing staff.

90Y offers a number of theoretical advantages over 131I, although the radioisotopes have not been directly compared conjugated to the same mAb. 90Y is a pure β emitter delivering higher energy radiation (2.3 MeV versus 0.6 MeV) at a longer path length (5.3 mm versus 0.8 mm). This increased path length would be expected to enhance the 'cross-fire effect' and could therefore potentially be advantageous in treating larger tumours, less well vascularized tumour nodules or tumours with heterogeneous antigen expression[33]. This longer path length is likely, however, to increase the normal tissue dose when targeting microscopic disease for which the shorter path length of 131I may be preferable. The half-life of 64 hours matches the biological half-life of murine mAbs and the absence of penetrating γ emissions enables delivery as an outpatient[28]. In addition, if a cell internalizes 90Y, it is likely to be retained within the cell[34]. In contrast if 131I conjugates are internalized by a cell they will be rapidly dehalogenated and the small 131I products rapidly released into the blood stream, reducing desired tumour absorbed radiation dose and increasing normal tissue exposure to radiation[35].

The major disadvantages of ^{90}Y relate to its greater expense, relatively limited availability and requirement for chelation radiochemistry making radiolabelling a more difficult procedure as high labelling efficiency of direct radiolabelling to the mAb is not achievable. In addition as ^{90}Y is a pure β-emitter, in the absence of γ emissions, there is a need to use a surrogate isotope ^{111}In to obtain images for biodistribution and dosimetry studies.

^{186}Re and ^{67}Cu have physical and chemical properties that make them attractive alternatives however their current limited availability has meant that these radioisotopes have received limited clinical use[36]. ^{211}At is an α emitter producing a particle of very high energy but with a very short path length. The high linear energy transfer radiation of α emitters may be lethal to cells with a single hits; however, the very short path length means that the isotope must be internalized to be effective and is likely to have little or no 'cross-fire' effect. The suitability of α emitters therefore appears limited to readily accessible tumours such as leukaemia cells in blood or bone marrow. The short half-life of about 7 hours complicates administration meaning that such radioisotopes are likely to require generation on the same site as delivery in the clinic. Despite this logistical hurdle, early clinical data in the treatment of leukaemia appear extremely promising[37,38]. Recent experimental RIT studies involving animal leukaemia models have also demonstrated the therapeutic potential of another α emitter, ^{213}Bi[39,40]. Recently, Oh *et al.* reported impressive therapeutic effects using an Auger emitter, ^{125}I-labelled mAb targeting on a tumour blood vessel (endothelial cell) specific protein, anti-Annex A1 to treat lung tumour-bearing rats[41].

7.3.2 Pre-dosing of monoclonal antibody in radioimmunotherapy

There are several factors that may theoretically limit lymphoma targeting of radiolabelled pan-B-cell mAb in RIT and these include:

1. complex formation of administered antibody with free circulating target antigen;

2. cross-reactivity with antigen-positive circulating lymphoma cells, normal B cells in the blood or spleen, or non-lymphoid tissues;

3. non-antigenic binding of antibody, such as binding by Fc arm of mAb.

In order to improve the biodistribution of radiolabelled mAb in RIT, it has become the established practice in clinical RIT targeting the CD20 antigen to give a pre-dose of unlabelled anti-CD20 mAb prior to the therapeutic dose of radioimmunoconjuagates[30,42]. The pre-dose is thought to prolong the circulating half-life of the radiolabelled mAb and thus increase the tumour retention of the labelled mAb by blocking 'non-specific' binding sites such as circulating and splenic B cells. However, increasingly larger dose of cold pre-dose of mAb pose at least a theoretical risk of blocking tumour antigen-binding sites and may therefore decrease the tumour uptake of radiolabelled mAb. In all of the initial registration studies, large amounts of unlabelled mAb (250 mg/m^2 rituximab) prior to ^{90}Y-ibritumomab tiuxetan and 450 mg tositumomab prior to ^{131}I-tositumomab, were given prior to the dosimetric studies and the larger therapeutic dose of a radioimmunconjugates (see Table 7.5).

Table 7.5 Pre-dose schedules for Zevalin^{TM} and Bexxar^{TM} RIT regimens

	Day 0 Dosimetric step	Days 0–7	Day 7 Therapeutic step
Bexxar^{TM}	**Pre-dose: tositumomab** 450 mg (60 min i.v. infusion)	Serial γ – camera imaging/counting for dosimetric assessment	Pre-dose: tositumomab 450 mg (60 min i.v. infusion)
	Dosimetric dose: ^{131}I-tositumomab 35 mg mAb containing ^{131}I 185 MBq (20 min i.v. infusion)		Therapeutic dose: ^{131}I-tositumomab 35 mg mAb containing ^{131}I activity to deliver 65–75 cGy total body dose (20 min i.v. infusion)
Zevalin^{TM}	**Pre-dose: rituximab** 250 mg/m^2 (60 min i.v. infusion)		Pre-dose: rituximab 250 mg/m^2 (60 min i.v. infusion)
	Dosimetric dose: ^{111}In-ibritumomab tuxetan 1.6 mg ibritumomab tiuxetan containing ^{111}In 185 MBq (10 min i.v. infusion)		Therapeutic dose: ^{90}Y-ibritumomab tiuxetan 3.2 mg ibritumomab tiuxetan containing ^{90}Y 14.8 MBq/kg or 11.1 MBq/kg for patients with platelet counts higher or lower than 150×10^9/l (10 min i.v. infusion)

The studies upon which the amount of mAb protein pre-dose or 'cold' or unlabelled mAb were established were, however, based on small patient numbers[43]. The dose of 250 mg/m^2 rituximab prior to ^{90}Y-ibritumomab tiuxetan was based on data from only six patients, and just three patients received 125 mg/m^2 and a further three patients the 250 mg/m^2 dose. The biodistribution was the same for both the 125 mg/m^2 and the 250 mg/m^2 dose, but the larger dose was chosen because of the encouraging single agent efficacy of rituximab. It was thought that the larger dose of rituximab might contribute to the overall efficacy of the ^{90}Y-ibritumomab treatment schedule[44].

The amount of mAb protein administered as the radioimmunoconjugate is considerably smaller than the large pre-doses of mAb in both ^{90}Y-ibritumomab tiuxetan and ^{131}I-tositumomab regimens. Just 3.2 mg of ibritumomab is used following the 250 mg/m^2 pre-dose of rituximab in the ^{90}Y-ibritumomab tiuxetan, whereas for ^{131}I-tositumomab 35 mg is given as ^{131}I-tositumomab following 450 mg of cold pre-dose of tositumomab[30,31,45,46]. In the registration studies for both ^{90}Y-ibritumomab tiuxetan, the pre-doses were given prior to both the dosimetric study and the therapeutic infusion, respectively. For ^{90}Y-ibritumomab tiuxetan within the EU there is no requirement for imaging whereas in the US this still forms part of the licensing agreement.

Both ^{90}Y-labelled ibritumomab tiuxetan and ^{131}I-labelled tositumomab are murine in origin. Murine mAb were initially the preferred option in the development of RIT reagents as it was hypothesized that the short half-life of a murine mAb was preferable to a chimeric or humanized mAb where by virtue of the human Fc arm the radioimmunoconjugate would have a substantially increased circulating half-life and thus lead to an increased exposure and overall radiation dose to bone marrow resulting in increased myelotoxicity[28]. Recent data have, however, suggested that this hypothesis may be incorrect and that the use radiolabelled chimeric mAb may not lead to increased myelotoxicity[47].

An accurate estimation of bone marrow dosimetry has proven to be extremely difficult practically because of the irregular distribution of active bone marrow involvement of tumour cells and diminished healthy bone marrow in previously heavily treated patients[48]. Wiseman and colleagues[49] used ^{111}In ibritumomab as a surrogate for ^{90}Y-ibritumomab in the dosimetric studies and failed to find any correlation between bone marrow dosimetry and myelotoxicity. Instead these workers found that simple clinical parameters such as weight of patient, baseline platelet count, and number of lines prior to therapy were more strongly correlated to myelotoxicity than was the bone marrow dosimetry. Wiseman *et al.* therefore argue that these inaccuracies mean that bone marrow dosimetry is not required and that ^{90}Y-ibritumomab can be give safely without dosimetry. The lack of correlation between the biodistribution of the radionuclide and haematological toxicity led to ^{90}Y-ibritumomab being approved within the EU without the necessity for imaging studies. In contrast, Wahl and colleagues have argued that patient-specific dosimetry as used in the ^{131}I-tositumomab treatment regimen achieves significantly better tumour dosimetry[31,42,49].

Further research is required to standardize the dosimetric methodology and studies with larger number of patients are likely to be helpful in further clarifying this issue. Most recently Dewaraja et al. reported that in comparison with their improved patient-specific, three-dimensional methods for SPECT reconstruction and absorbed dose calculation, the currently widely used conventional clinical RIT dosimetry calculation protocol could have substantially underestimated the radiation doses delivered to tumours by RIT especially for smaller tumours[50]. In their report, they found that the mean tumour absorbed dose estimate from the improved calculation protocol was 7% higher than that from conventional dosimetry. Aside from the biological factors and dosimetry methodology factors mentioned above, the intrinsic physical properties of current Gamma camera/SPECT facilities used in such dosimetry studies have spatial resolution limited to about 0.8 cm. This degree of resolution makes it unlikely that a gamma camera image can accurately reflect the real distribution of infused mAb within a targeted tumour or normal organ at a microscopic level and be able to accurately measure the heterogeneity of the radiation dose.

7.3.3 Treatment dosing schedule

RIT with ^{90}Y-ibritumomab tiuxetan is completed within 1 week and consists of a single dose of the therapeutic radioimmunoconjugate. Treatment schedule includes intravenous infusion of rituximab (250 mg/m^2) on days 1 and 8[44]. As ^{90}Y is a pure β emitter to facilitate gamma camera imaging ^{111}In is used as a surrogate and chelated to ibritumomab tiuxetan for dosimetry. Imaging was done as part of the registration studies on day 1 [at a dose of 185 MBq (5 mCi)] following the rituximab infusion with imaging done at 2–24 hours, at 48–72 hours, and at 90–120 hours postinjection and two scans still form part of the approved schedule within the US[45]. ^{90}Y-ibritumomab tiuxetan is administered within 4 hours after the second rituximab infusion via slow intravenous push over a period of 10 minutes provided a 0.2 or 0.22 μm low protein binding filter is in place.

An initial phase I dose escalation study of ^{90}Y-ibritumomab tiuxetan up to a myeloablative activity of 1850 MBq (50 mCi), that included 14 patients with relapsed or refractory low- or intermediate-grade B-cell NHL established that pre-dosing with the unlabelled ibritumomab (murine antibody) improved the tumour dose and also demonstrated that the haematological toxicity was correlated most closely with body weight, rather than body surface area[51]. A further phase I/II study was subsequently performed and this demonstrated that the biodistribution of the radioimmunoconjugate can be improved by pre-dosing with rituximab (chimeric antibody) and no difference was found between 125 mg/m^2 or the 250 mg/m^2 dose. Myelotoxicity was found to be the dose-limiting toxicity and the maximum tolerated dose (MTD) was identified as 14.8 MBq/kg or 0.4 mCi/kg (to a maximum dose of 1 184 MBq or 32 mCi) for patients with a baseline platelet count of $\geq$150 000 $\times$ 10^9/l and 11.1 MBq/kg or 0.3 mCi/kg for patients with baseline platelet counts of <150 000 $\times$ 10^9/l l but $\geq$100 000 $\times$ 10^9/l[44]. Another study specifically examined the tolerability of a reduced dose in patients with mild thrombocytopenia (baseline platelet count of 100–150 000 $\times$ 10^9/l). This study demonstrated that such patients can be safely treated with ^{90}Y-ibritumomab tiuxetan at a dose of 11.1 MBq/kg or 0.3 mCi/kg[52].

The ^{131}I-tositumomab therapeutic regimen differs from ^{90}Y-ibritumomab tiuxetan in that it is completed in four visits over 1–2 weeks as shown in Table 7.6. This regimen involves an initial biodistribution/dosimetry study followed by a therapeutic infusion given 7–14 days later, which requires a 4–6-day inpatient stay in Europe. The legislation for radiation protection differs substantially in the USA from state to state and the same Bexxar schedule

Table 7.6 Bexxar™ (^{131}I-tositumomab) therapeutic regimen

	Dosimetric step		Therapeutic step
Day 0	Days 2, 3, or 4	Day 6 or 7	Days 7–14
Tositumomab 450 mg (60 min i.v. infusion)	Gamma camera count 2 (post-urination)	Gamma camera count 3 (post-urination)	Tositumomab 450 mg (60 min i.v. infusion)
^{131}I-tositumomab 35 mg mAb containing ^{131}I 185 MBq (20 min i.v. infusion)			^{131}I-tositumomab 35 mg mAb containing ^{131}I activity to deliver 65–75 cGy total body dose (20 min i.v. infusion)
Gamma camera count 1 (prior to urination)			Thyroid protection medication for 14 days

has been routinely given requiring an overnight stay or even as an outpatient in some states.

Each infusion of the ^{131}I-tositumomab is preceded by an infusion of a pre-dose of 450 mg 'cold' or unlabelled tositumomab. Whole body gamma camera imaging is performed three times over the week following the trace-labelled infusion to calculate the whole body half-time and the dose required for the therapeutic infusion to deliver 65–75 cGy of whole body irradiation (usually 100–150 mCi)[53]. A therapeutic total body dose of 75 cGy was preceded by a dosimetric step. Dose adjustments to 65 cGy were made for a baseline platelet count of 100 000/mm^3 to <150 000/mm^3 and for obesity.

7.4 Precautions and side-effects in use

Successful implementation of RIT requires a multidisciplinary approach, which ideally includes haematologists/oncologists, nuclear medicine physicians, physicists, radiopharmacists, and trained nursing staff. Regular communication between the haematology/oncology department and the nuclear medicine department is essential throughout treatment. For the successful delivery of RIT a co-ordinator is required to organize the logistics of delivering RIT. An experienced haematologist/oncologist is usually responsible for evaluating patients, determining eligibility for RIT, obtaining informed consent and pre-dosing with 'cold' or unlabelled mAb, providing the appropriate supportive care and safety monitoring required for mAb infusions. Good practice should involve the patients who are being considered for treatment consulting with the nuclear medicine physician or radiation oncologist (radioisotope delivery certificate holder) prior to the treatment to confirm that all safety criteria for treatment are met and to provide the patient with additional information regarding radiation safety issues and the practicalities of RIT. The certificate holder (nuclear medicine physician/radiation oncologist) is responsible for the preparation and administration of RIT.

For the preparation of ^{90}Y-ibritumomab tiuxetan only trained personnel should perform the labelling of ibritumomab tiuxetan with radiopharmaceutical grade ^{90}Y, with appropriate facilities for shielding, calibration, and quality control. Emitted β particles are completely absorbed by plastic or acrylic pot with a thickness of 1 cm. Calibration methods are included in the package insert provided with the ^{90}Y-ibritumomab tiuxetan preparation kit. In terms of quality control a radioincorporation assay to determine radiochemical purity should be performed. To ensure the accuracy of results, all quality control testing should be performed in duplicates, and the ^{90}Y-ibritumomab tiuxetan preparation should not be administered if radiochemical purity is <95%.

^{131}I-tositumomab is delivered radiolabelled and the appropriate quality control, which includes measurements of labelling efficiency and immunoreactivity have been performed at the production facility prior to dispatch. The patient specific dose has been calculated from the whole body dosimetry and pre-ordered and therefore only the required activity of ^{131}I-tositumomab requires measurement prior to administration.

Both ^{131}I-tositumomab and ^{90}Y-ibritumomab tiuxetan should be administered through a patent indwelling cannula, with a 0.20–0.22 micron in-line filter placed between the injection port and the patient. Once ^{90}Y-ibritumomab tiuxetan has been made up it should be administered no later than 8 hours after preparation. The use of a remote infusion system is recommended for the delivery of both radioimmunoconjuagates, and the line should be flushed with normal saline solution to ensure that all medication has been administered to the patient. Residual activity in the syringe and tubing should then be measured. Acute side-effects during the infusion of the radioimmunoconjuagates are extremely rare, but steroids and antihistamines should be readily available during ^{131}I-tositumomab and ^{90}Y-ibritumomab tiuxetan administration. If extravasation occurs, the infusion should be stopped immediately, and the arm should be elevated and massaged to facilitate lymphatic drainage.

Patients can be reassured that they pose a negligible radiation risk to their family and close friends once discharged as an outpatient after receiving ^{90}Y-ibritumomab. On discharge, patients should be advised to wash their hands thoroughly after urination (male patients should urinate seated), clear up spilled urine or blood immediately and use condoms for sexual intercourse for at least 1 week following treatment. As with other cancer treatments, effective contraception for up to a whole year after treatment (to avoid pregnancy) is recommended for both male and female patients. For women, it is very unlikely that fertility will be affected, while men may experience a temporary loss of fertility. On rare occasions, radiation may cause permanent sterility in men and therefore for male patients who remain keen to father children cryopreservation of semen should be considered as a precaution.

Myelosuppression was found to be the dose-limiting toxicity of RIT for both ^{90}Y-ibritumomab tiuxetan and ^{131}I-tositumomab. An analysis of all patients treated in ^{90}Y-ibritumomab tiuxetan trials ($n = 261$) indicated that 28% will experience grade 4 neutropenia and 8% will experience grade 4 thrombocytopenia[54].

Safety data for ^{90}Y-ibritumomab tiuxetan from four clinical trials were reviewed retrospectively in an integrated analysis[46] encompassing 349 patients of whom 345 patients (99%) completed treatment. Although 80% of patients reported non-haematological adverse events (AEs), those were generally mild to moderate in severity with asthenia, nausea, and chills being the most common events that were considered probably or possibly related to treatment. Only 11% (39 patients) of all patients experienced grade 3–4 non-haematological toxicity.

The primary and dose-limiting toxicity associated with ^{90}Y-ibritumomab tiuxetan was transient, reversible myelosuppression, typically developing delayed by week 4–6 reaching nadirs by week 7–9. Of note, thrombocytopenia grade 1–2 and 3–4 occurred in 37% and 63% of patients, respectively. Eighty-seven per cent of patients with grade 3–4 thrombocytopenia recovered to >50 000/μl by week 12 following therapy. Grade 3–4 neutropenia was observed in 30% of patients, with 90% recovering to >1000/μl within 12 weeks post-treatment. For patients, who received growth factor support with filgastrim the median duration of neutropenia was reduced from 27 to 19 days. Grade 3 and 4 anaemia developed in 13% and 4% of patients, respectively. Of all patients, 22% required platelet transfusions and 20% required red blood cell transfusions.

Incidences of severe thrombocytopenia and neutropenia correlated significantly with degree of bone marrow involvement and platelet counts at baseline, underscoring the importance of excluding patients with >25% bone marrow infiltration and inadequate bone marrow reserve. Patients who had more than two prior chemotherapies were twice as likely to develop grade 4 thrombocytopenia, whereas number of prior chemotherapies did not correlate with longer median duration of neutropenia, thrombocytopenia, and anaemia.

It is important that patients and treating physicians are aware of the delayed haematological toxicity for both ^{90}Y-ibritumomab tiuxetan and also for ^{131}I-tositumomab and the necessity for mandatory blood count monitoring from 3 weeks after RIT performed at least once weekly until haematological recovery, which is usually at about 10–12 weeks post-RIT. If the blood count monitoring is to be done by a clinician other than the physician in charge of delivering the RIT, clear instructions are required regarding the nature of the delayed nadir and the requirement for appropriate haematological supportive care.

For ^{90}Y-ibritumomab tiuxetan the total number of B cells and levels of IgM were found to decline after treatment but to have recovered after 6–9 months. The median T-cell counts and levels of IgG and IgA remained stable following treatment with ^{90}Y-ibritumomab tiuxetan. Most importantly treatment with ^{90}Y-ibritumomab tiuxetan was not associated with an excess rate of infections. In fact, incidence of infectious complications was low with upper respiratory and urinary tract infections occurring in 5% and 7% of patients, respectively. Only 8% of all patients received antibiotic therapy during the treatment period.

No significant difference in the incidence of haematological and non-haematological grade 3–4 AEs was observed in patients >65 years as compared with younger patients. Despite concerns about the potential of an increased risk of radiation-induced secondary haematological malignancies, the observed rate of secondary myelodysplastic syndromes (MDS) and acute leukaemias was <1% (5/348), comparable with a similar patient population treated with alkylating agents[55].

The radiation dosimetry studies demonstrated that the administration of ^{90}Y-ibritumomab tiuxetan results in minimal radiation exposure to non-targeted organs, with the largest radiation dose delivered to the spleen (median absorbed dose, 848 cGy)[45]. Low levels of Bremmstrahlung radiation are expected with ^{90}Y-ibritumomab tiuxetan, therefore a study was conducted to determine the radiation dose absorbed by family members of patients receiving ^{90}Y-ibritumomab tiuxetan at a dose of 14.8 MBq/kg (0.4 mCi/kg) body weight. In this study, the family member who was likely to have the closest contact with the patient during the 7-day period following treatment wore an electronic personal dosimeter, and an ion chamber was used to measure radiation exposure at a distance of 1 meter from the low chest of patients immediately after ^{90}Y-ibritumomab tiuxetan administration. The median deep-dose equivalent radiation exposure reached a total accumulation of 0.035 mSv over the 7-day study period (range, 0.014–0.079), while the median radiation exposure at a 1-meter distance from the patient was 0.00295 mSv/hour (range, 0.0024–0.0039 mSv/hour). Thus, the investigators concluded that the risk of radiation exposure to family members was extremely low and in the same range as background radiation[56].

For ^{131}I-tositumomab the short-term non-haematological AEs are also generally mild, and include typically fatigue, nausea, fever, vomiting, pruritus, and rash, which usually respond well to antihistamines. Hypothyroidism appears one of the most notable long-term adverse effects after ^{131}I-labelled mAb treatment, which can, however, be easily managed with thyroid hormone replacement. Most recently, Zelenetz reviewed the multicentre RIT trials using ^{131}I-tositumomab in NHL patients and reported that elevated thyroid-stimulating hormone was observed in five of 59 patients in the phase I study[58]. However, Liu *et al.* observed elevated thyroid-stimulating hormone in 59% of patients treated in Seattle with myeloablative dose of ^{131}I-tositumomab[59]. HAMA reactions appear to be substantially lower in previously treated NHL patients compared with the rates experienced in

Table 7.7 Radiation dose estimates for patients treated with ^{90}Y-ibritumomab tiuxetan[57]

Organ	n	Total dose (cGy)	
		Median	Range
Red marrow	72	70.6	17.5–221
Bone surfaces	72	60.1	19.9–157
Kidneys	72	15.4	0.27–76
Liver	72	532	234–1856
Lungs	72	216	93.6–457
Spleen	66*	848	76–1902
Urinary bladder wall	72	95.4	44.4–270
Total body	72	59.5	23.4–79.3
Other organs†	72	43.5	12.5–58.5

* Six patients had prior splenectomies.

†Includes adrenals, brain, breasts, gallbladder wall, heart wall, lower large intestine wall, muscle, pancreas, skin, small intestine, stomach, thymus, thyroid, upper large intestine wall, and ovaries and uterus (female) or testes (male).

solid tumour RIT[15]. DeNardo *et al.* analysed 617 samples from 112 subjects, including 85 patients with B-cell malignancies. They found that 77% of B-cell malignancy patients developed no response or a weak response after multiple doses of mouse Lym-1 antibody[60]. In a separate study, Zelenetz observed similar results with approximately 10% of ^{131}I-tositumomab treated patients developed positive HAMA reaction. However, in the recently published study involving previously untreated follicular lymphoma patients, Kaminski *et al.* reported 48 of 76 (63%) patients developed detectable HAMA after a single course of treatment with ^{131}I-labelled tositumomab[14].

Secondary malignancy following RIT has fortunately proved to be rare[14,58]. Recently 1071 RIT-treated patients were assessed for treatment-related MDS and acute myeloid leukaemia (AML). Among them, 995 patients with low grade and transformed low-grade NHL had been treated with a median of three previous therapies (range, 1–13 therapies) prior to RIT. Seventy-six patients received RIT as their initial therapy for follicular NHL. For the previously treated patients, the median follow-up from the diagnosis of NHL and RIT was 6 years and 2 years, respectively; for the patients who received RIT as their initial therapy, the corresponding median follow-up times were 5.6 years and 4.6 years, respectively. Of the 995 previously treated patients, 35 (3.5%) cases of treatment-related MDS/AML were reported and

13 cases were confirmed to have developed MDS/AML following RIT. This incidence was found to be consistent with that expected on the basis of patients' prior chemotherapy for NHL. With a median follow-up approaching 5 years, no case of treatment-related MDS/AML has been reported in the 76 patients receiving ^{131}I-tositumomab as their initial therapy[61]. Administration of the ^{131}I-labelled tositumomab therapeutic regimen results in sustained depletion of circulating CD20-positive cells. The impact of administration of the ^{131}I-labelled tositumomab therapeutic regimen on circulating CD20-positive cells was assessed in two clinical studies, one conducted in chemotherapy naive patients and one in heavily pretreated patients. The assessment of circulating lymphocytes did not distinguish normal from malignant cells. Consequently, assessment of recovery of normal B-cell function was not directly assessed. Lymphocyte recovery began at approximately 12 weeks following treatment. Among patients who had CD20-positive cell counts recorded at baseline and at 6 months, eight of 58 (14%) chemotherapy naive patients had CD20-positive cell counts below normal limits at 6 months and six of 19 (32%) heavily pretreated patients had CD20-positive cell counts below normal limits at 6 months. There was no consistent effect of the ^{131}I-labelled tositumomab therapeutic regimen on post-treatment serum IgG, IgA, or IgM levels.

Estimations of radiation-absorbed doses for ^{131}I-tositumomab were performed using sequential whole body images and the MIRDOSE 3 software program. Patients with apparent thyroid, stomach, or intestinal imaging were selected for organ dosimetry analyses. The estimated radiation-absorbed doses to organs and marrow from a course of the ^{131}I-labelled tositumomab therapeutic regimen are presented in Table 7.8.

As regards the immediate follow-up post-RIT and beyond it is strongly recommended that the haematologist/oncologist is responsible for the post-treatment evaluation of the patient, keeping the nuclear medicine physician informed about the patient's progress. Follow-up involves weekly full blood count from 3 weeks following RIT until haematological recovery. Response to treatment should be assessed no earlier than 3 months after treatment, and even at this point clinicians should be aware that the quality of response may continue to improve beyond this time with the conversion of PRs to CRs occurring many weeks and months later in some patients.

7.5 Clinical efficacy of radioimmunotherapy in non-Hodgkin lymphoma

Although clinical RIT trials in NHL differ in terms of eligibility criteria, antibody, and radioisotopes used, dose, number of treatments, doses of

Table 7.8 Estimated radiation-absorbed organ doses for ^{131}I-tositumomab

	^{131}I-labelled tositumomab	
	mGy/MBq Median	mGy/MBq Range
From organ regions of interest (ROIs)		
Thyroid	2.71	1.4–6.2
Kidneys	1.96	1.5–2.5
ULI wall	1.34	0.8–1.7
LLI wall	1.30	0.8–1.6
Heart wall	1.25	0.5–1.8
Spleen	1.14	0.7–5.4
Testes	0.83	0.3–1.3
Liver	0.82	0.6–1.3
Lungs	0.79	0.5–1.1
Red marrow	0.65	0.5–1.1
Stomach wall	0.40	0.2–0.8
From whole body ROIs		
Urine bladder wall	0.64	0.6–0.9
Bone surfaces	0.41	0.4–0.6
Pancreas	0.31	0.2–0.4
Gall bladder wall	0.29	0.2.- 0.3
Adrenals	0.28	0.2–0.3
Ovaries	0.25	0.2–0.3
Small intestine	0.23	0.2–0.3
Thymus	0.22	0.1–0.3
Uterus	0.20	0.2–0.2
Muscle	0.18	0.1–0.2
Breasts	0.16	0.1–0.2
Skin	0.13	0.1–0.2
Brain	0.13	0.1–0.2
Total body	0.24	0.2–0.3

unlabelled mAb pre-infused or co-infused, and the biodistribution or dosimetry estimations required for administration of a therapeutic dose of radiolabelled mAb, virtually all clinical studies performed to date have shown high response rates in for RIT in NHL[12,14,15,24,62,63].

DeNardo et al. initially pioneered RIT for NHL with ^{131}I-labelled anti-HLA-DR mAb (Lym-1)[33,64]. In their early studies, patients were given fractionated doses (30–60 mCi) of ^{131}I-labelled Lym-1 at 2–6-week intervals[65]. Thirty patients with relapsed NHL or chronic lymphocytic leukaemia were treated. Three (10%) achieved CR and 14 (47%) achieved PR for an overall response rate of 57%. A subsequent trial investigating the efficacy of escalating doses of ^{131}I-labelled Lym-1 (40–100 mCi/m²) achieved an overall response rate of 52% in 21-treatment courses administered to 20 patients, with seven patients (33%) achieved CR, four patients (19%) achieved PR[22]. Goldenberg et al. used ^{131}I-labelled anti-CD22 antibody (LL2) to treat a variety of B-cell lymphomas. In one of their trials, four of 17 patients achieved objective remission including 1 CR[17]. In another trial, ^{90}Y-labelled LL2 were administered to seven patients with B-cell lymphomas, two of whom achieved PR[66]. A recent dose-escalation trial reported nine of 20 assessable patients showing objective responses with two CR[67].

The clinical trials conducted in B-cell lymphomas that have resulted in the most impressive clinical results to date have come from the use radiolabelled anti-CD20 mAb. Kaminski and colleagues initially conducted a series of trials at the University of Michigan using the ^{131}I-tositumomab for the treatment of relapsed follicular lymphoma[14,23,43,68]. In the pivotal study a single treatment of ^{131}I-tositumomab was shown to provide vastly superior disease-free survival compared with the last qualifying chemotherapy in a group of 60 extensively pretreated patients whereby the response to ^{131}I-tositumomab was compared with their previous response to chemotherapy in the same group of patients follicular or transformed follicular lymphoma[23]. On the basis of these clinical trials, ^{131}I-tositumomab was belatedly approved by the US FDA in June 2003[69].

Since 1990 over 800 patients with 'low-grade' and transformed lymphoma have been treated with ^{131}I-tositumomab. Long-term follow-up data was presented at the American Society of Haematology Annual Meeting (ASH) 2002 on 250 of these patients indicating a response rate of 56% with 30% of patients achieving a CR. Perhaps the most impressive fact was that 70% of the patients who achieved a CR are alive and remain in CR at up to 7.8 years with a median follow-up of almost 4 years[70]. An analysis of prognostic factors has confirmed that this remarkable durability of response cannot be accounted for by patient selection in the reported trials[71]. Of the patients that achieved CR, 89% had stage III/IV disease, 32% had no response to their last therapy, 45% had more than four prior therapies, 50% had bulky disease, and 43% had bone marrow involvement.

Impressive response rates have also been seen in patients that were refractory to rituximab. Horning and colleagues have treated 40 patients with low-grade NHL, 72% of which had received four or more previous lines of therapy and 60 % of which had failed to respond to rituximab. An overall response rate of 68% with a CR rate of 30% was noted and a median duration of response of 14.7 months reported. Nine of the 12 complete responders remained in CR at the time of presentation with a range of 12–26 months[72]. More recently an analysis including 230 patients treated with ^{131}I-tositumomab was made. Independently assessed durable CRs were noted with similar frequency in patients with rituximab-refractory disease (28%) and rituximab naive patients all of which had chemotherapy refractory disease (23%). With a median follow-up of 4.6 years, 75% of patients continue in CR[73].

Highly promising results have also been seen in the frontline treatment of previously untreated low-grade lymphomas using ^{131}I-tositumomab. The most recent update included 76 patients with a median follow-up of 5.1 years. An encouraging overall response rate of 95% was seen with 75% achieving CR. The actuarial 5-year progression-free survival for all patients was 59%, with a median progression-free survival of 6.1 years. Haematological toxicity was moderate, with no patient requiring transfusion or haematopoietic growth factors[14,70,74].

A total of four clinical trials, including three phase I/II and one randomized study formed the basis of the FDA submission for ^{90}Y-ibritumomab tiuxetan. The randomized controlled trial compared ^{90}Y-ibritumomab tiuxetan with rituximab in relapsed or refractory low-grade B-cell NHL and the results demonstrated for the first time that RIT can lead to superior overall and CR rates to those seen with 'naked' mAb[11]. Seventy-three patients received two doses of rituximab 250 mg/m^2 a week apart as pre-dosing followed by a single dose of ^{90}Y-ibritumomab tiuxetan 0.4 mCi/kg body weight. Seventy patients in the control arm received rituximab 375 mg/m^2 weekly for 4 weeks. The overall response rate was 80% for the labelled antibody group versus 56% for the rituximab alone group ($P = 0.002$). CR rates were 30% and 16% in the ^{90}Y-ibritumomab tiuxetan and rituximab groups respectively. Subsequent longer-term analysis of these initial registration studies revealed that ^{90}Y-ibritumomab tiuxetan appears able to deliver durable remissions and for those patients that achieved a CR, the median duration of response approached 4 years and ongoing responses of more than 4 years have been reported[54,75].

Clinical responses have also been observed for ^{90}Y-ibritumomab tiuxetan in transformed follicular and relapsed diffuse large B-cell lymphoma (DLBC). Within the initial Phase I/II study reported a response rate of 58% with a 33% CR rate in a group of just 12 patients that had relapsed following two previous chemotherapy regimens that included CHOP[75,76]. A prospective, single-arm, open-label, non-randomized, multicentre phase II trial was therefore undertaken to evaluate the efficacy and safety of ^{90}Y-ibritumomab tiuxetan in patients >60 years of age with relapsed or primary refractory DLBCL not appropriate for autologous stem cell transplantation. Patients were divided into two groups with first those previously treated with chemotherapy alone (Group A, $n = 76$) and secondly those previously treated with chemotherapy and rituximab (Group B, $n = 28$)[77].

All patients received a single dose of 14.8 MBq/kg (0.4 mCi/kg) ^{90}Y-ibritumomab tiuxetan up to a maximum dose of 1184 MBq/kg (32 mCi). In total, 103 patients were evaluable for efficacy, and 104 for safety. An overall response rate (ORR) of 44% was observed in the entire study population. In Group A, the ORR was over 50 %. In Group B, where 37% of patients were refractory to rituximab-CHOP, the ORR was 19%. AEs, with the exception of haematological AEs were generally mild (grade 1/2). The incidence of severe infection was low, with only 7% of patients hospitalized for infection during the study. The results of this study were encouraging and clinical trials are now underway in the USA or at an advanced stage of development in the EU to integrate ^{90}Y-ibritumomab tiuxetan into the front line treatment of DLBC alongside rituximab chemotherapy schedules.

Although no comparative clinical trial has been performed between ^{90}Y-ibritumomab tiuxetan and ^{131}I-tositumomab and such a study is unlikely ever to be done, the two drugs appear from the published results to have very similar response rates and response durations. The integration of ^{90}Y-ibritumomab tiuxetan and ^{131}I-tositumomab into routine clinical practice is likely therefore to depend on the cost and convenience of each therapy rather than perceived differences in clinical efficacy. However, the radiation protection issues may make the extra expense of ^{90}Y worthwhile, as the necessity for 5–6 days in-patient stay for patients (within the EU) receiving ^{131}I-tositumomab may influence clinicians on health economic grounds. In addition the removal of the dosimetric dose, within the EU, simplifies the delivering of ^{90}Y-ibritumomab tiuxetan as recent studies have failed to demonstrate a consistent correlation between the estimated bone marrow dose and toxicity but have shown that ^{90}Y-ibritumomab tiuxetan can be safely prescribed according to body weight and platelet count[30,49].

7.6 **Alternative treatments and relative efficacy of radioisotope therapy**

Although RIT has emerged an effective treatment for NHL, the underlying mechanisms of action and in particular the interaction of irradiation and mAb in RIT are still poorly understood[28,78,79]. To further optimize RIT in lymphoma there remain, a number of important questions where further work is required to address such issues as: (a) whether a radiation dose response exists in RIT of lymphoma; (b) the requirement and the usefulness of dosimetry for predicting tumour responses and/or normal tissue toxicity; and (c) how best to integrate RIT in the treatment algorithms for NHL.

The estimation of the radiation absorbed dose has been an essential part of evaluating risks and benefits associated with conventional radiotherapy and it is vital in treatment planning, predicting radiation effects, correcting biological effects with dose, and maintaining complete patient records. One of the fundamental potential advantages of RIT is the ability to deliver higher targeted radiation dose to the tumour than to normal tissue and thus enhance the specific tumour killing. The fact that radioisotopes emit ionizing radiation not only enables them to be used in therapy but also to be quantified using radiation dosimetry. However, due to the relative complexity of the radiation dose estimation for RIT, the clinical importance of dosimetry in RIT of NHL currently remains controversial. While some investigators regard dosimetry an essential component of RIT practice, others do not think it necessary[80–83].

Gamma camera imaging takes advantage of the emitted γ radiation from γ emitting radioisotopes and enables patient dosimetric assessments. The distribution of radioactivity in the body or in individual source organs can be roughly determined by sequential imaging using planar scintillation cameras or tomographic single photon emission computed tomography (SPECT). Using conjugate imaging data with patient body weight, organ volumetrics, blood sampling, urine sampling, marrow biopsy, the patient dosimetry can be estimated[17,48,66]. The MIRD (Medical Internal Radiation Dose) committee developed a dedicated computer-based program MIRDOSE to fulfil this task and this program is widely used in clinical RIT trials.

To date despite the high response rates seen in RIT of lymphoma clinical dosimetry studies have thus far failed to show a consistent dose–response relationship[15]. More recently, the Michigan group have concluded that there is a radiation dose–response at least for ^{131}I-tositumomab[42,80]. However, their conclusions are not shared by other investigators in the field[82,83]. Postema argues that none of the RIT dosing methods use tumour dosimetry to determine the dose administered to patients because the myelotoxicity of radiolabelled mAb will limit the increments of radioactivity dose, but not the tumour absorbed dose[82]. More recently, Goldenberg and colleagues commented that because RIT has two potentially therapeutic arms, namely radiation and mAb mechanisms, poor radiation targeting dose may not exclude good therapeutic response from the mAb[83].

There is now substantial evidence that mAb are an active component of RIT and that mAb effector mechanisms are important. Therefore, it is possible that in the evaluation of RIT radiation dose response, the mAb effector mechanisms may help to explain the conflicting data regarding the correlation between tumour dosimetry and therapeutic results. Although the exact *in vivo* mechanisms of tumour killing by anti-CD20 mAb remain incompletely understood, pre-clinical data have suggested that the action of rituximab may include antibody-dependent cellular cytotoxicity, complement-dependent cytotoxicity (CDC), and the direct induction of apoptosis through cell surface mediated signalling transduction[84].

Cragg and Glennie[85] reported that a panel of anti-CD20 mAbs (rituximab, ibritumomab, 1F5 and anti-B1) act through distinctively different mechanisms in the therapy of two lymphoma xenograft models. Rituximab and 1F5 redistribute CD20 into membrane rafts, are bound efficiently by the complement component C1q and deposit C3b resulting in CDC, which forms the major therapeutic effect of these two mAbs. In contrast, complement depletion had no effect on the potent therapeutic activity of anti-B1 (tositumomab), a mAb that does not redistribute CD20 into membrane rafts, bind C1q or cause efficient CDC. $F(ab')_2$ fragments of anti-B1 (tositumomab) but not 1F5 were observed able to provide substantial immunotherapy, indicating that non-Fc-dependent mechanisms are involved in the tositumomab action. In accordance with this, tositumomab was shown to induce much higher levels of apoptosis than rituximab and 1F5, suggesting that, while complement is important for the action of rituximab and 1F5, this is not the case for tositumomab, which more likely functions through its ability to induce downstream signal transduction that results in apoptosis. So far, clinical results concerning the mechanisms of action of anti-CD20 mAbs has been controversial and there remains considerable uncertainty. While some of the investigators addressed the importance of CDC in clinical immunotherapy, others have found that it fails to predict the therapeutic response[86,87].

The contribution of targeted radiation delivered by mAb to tumour responses has also been investigated. Over the last few years the addition of targeted radiation in RIT has demonstrated superior clinical responses to unlabelled mAb[11,12]. In a recently published multicentre, randomized study comparing treatment outcomes for unlabelled tositumomab (pre-dose) and ^{131}I-labelled tositumomab to an equivalent total dose of unlabelled tositumomab involving 78 patients with refractory/relapsed NHL (median follow-up 42.6 months), Davis *et al.* reported that responses in ^{131}I-labelled tositumomab versus unlabelled tositumomab groups. Overall response was 55% versus 19% ($P = 0.002$); CR 33% versus 8% ($P = 0.012$); median duration of overall response not reached versus 28.1 months; median duration of CR not reached in either arm; and median time to progression 6.3 versus 5.5 months ($P = 0.031$), respectively. Although haematological toxicity was more severe and non-haematological AEs were more frequent after ^{131}I-labelled tositumomab than after tositumomab alone, there were no serious infectious or bleeding complications. The frequency of developing HAMA was similar in the two arms with 27% (^{131}I-labelled tositumomab group) versus 19% (tositumomab alone group), respectively. This study demonstrated that although unlabelled tositumomab showed single agent activity, the conjugation of ^{131}I to tositumomab significantly enhanced the therapeutic efficacy[12].

Furthermore, the randomized study of ^{90}Y-ibritumomab tiuxetan versus rituximab confirmed the superior overall response rate (80%) of the RIT over the mAb alone (56%) ($P = 0.002$). CR were 30% and 16% in the ^{90}Y-labelled ibritumomab tiuxetan and rituximab groups respectively[11]. In conclusion, there is now good evidence to support the view that targeted radiation significantly enhances the response rate of the anti-CD20 mAb and that both targeted radiation and mAb effector mechanisms appear to play an important part in the high response rates seen in lymphoma.

The relative importance of mAb effector mechanisms and targeted radiation are difficult to measure and it is practically impossible to dissect the action of the two components in clinical RIT. Preclinical studies using well defined syngeneic animal models are therefore required to investigate this further and clarify the relative contributions of mAb effector mechanisms and targeted radiation[88]. Our group and others have investigated the relative contributions of antibody and targeted radiation to the clearance of tumour *in vivo*, using different syngeneic murine B-cell lymphoma models. Using a ^{131}I-anti-major histocompatibility class (MHC) II which was only effective in targeting radiation to tumour and where the anti-MHC II mAb has no therapeutic activity alone, we were able to investigate the role of targeted radiation alone and use additional mAb to look at mAb effector functions. When ^{131}I-anti-MHC II was used alone there were no long-term survivors as the radiation dose delivered was increased. In contrast, using the combination of ^{131}I-anti-MHC II in the presence of an unlabelled anti-idiotype (surface specific immunoglobulin or Id) a 100% disease free survival was found in two different B-cell lymphoma models at the higher radiation dose. Using *in vivo* tracking it was demonstrated that treatment with radiation plus anti-Id mAb resulted in a substantially greater reduction of tumour cells than with either treatment alone. Furthermore, prolonged survival could be achieved in these animal tumour models using ^{131}I-anti-MHC II in addition with other B-cell signalling mAb. Furthermore, the ability of some anti-B-cell mAb to improve survival with targeted radiotherapy appeared to correlate with their ability to initiate intracellular signal transduction. Together these data illustrate that using one mAb to target radiation to tumour and a second to induce cell signalling may be an effective new strategy in delivering RIT to lymphomas and enables more accurate estimations of the role of mAb and targeted radiation in the successful clearance of tumour.

In summary, mAb is highly likely to contribute to the treatment effects of RIT through its intrinsic therapeutic mechanisms. Preclinical work has indicated that the intrinsic cytotoxicity of mAb could be as important as its ability to effectively deliver targeted radiotherapy in the RIT of lymphoma[88,89]. Further investigation is, however, required to elucidate the mechanisms of the interaction between the mAb and low-dose rate irradiation. Such data may help to provide new insights into the mechanisms underlying successful RIT.

References

1. Fisher RI (2003). Overview of non-Hodgkin's lymphoma: biology, staging, and treatment. *Seminars in Oncology* **30**(2 Suppl. 4): 3–9.
2. Wingo PA, Tong T, Bolden S (1995). Cancer statistics, 1995. *CA: A Cancer Journal for Clinicians* **45**: 8–30.
3. Wingo PA, Ries LA, Rosenberg HM, Miller DS, Edwards BK (1998). Cancer incidence and mortality, 1973–1995: a report card for the US. *Cancer* **82**(6): 1197–207.
4. Weir HK, Thun MJ, Hankey BF, *et al.* (2003). Annual report to the nation on the status of cancer, 1975–2000, featuring the uses of surveillance data for cancer prevention and control. *Journal of the National Cancer Institute* **95**(17): 1276–99.
5. Armitage JO, Weisenburger DD (1998). New approach to classifying non-Hodgkin's lymphomas: clinical features of the major histologic subtypes. Non-Hodgkin's Lymphoma Classification Project. *Journal of Clinical Oncology* **16**(8): 2780–95.
6. Harris NL, Jaffe ES, Diebold J, *et al.* (1999). World Health Organization classification of neoplastic diseases of the hematopoietic and lymphoid tissues: report of the Clinical Advisory Committee meeting-Airlie House, Virginia, November 1997. *Journal of Clinical Oncology* **17**(12): 3835–49.
7. Kohler G, Milstein C (1975). Continuous cultures of fused cells secreting antibody of predefined specificity. *Nature* **256**(5517): 495–7.
8. Avivi I, Robinson S, Goldstone A (2003). Clinical use of rituximab in haematological malignancies. *British Journal of Cancer* **89**(8): 1389–94.

9. McLaughlin P (2001). Rituximab: perspective on single agent experience, and future directions in combination trials. *Critical Reviews in Oncology/Hematology* **40**: 3–16.

10. Coiffier B (2005). Monoclonal antibodies in the treatment of indolent lymphomas. *Best Practice and Research Clinical Haematology* **18**: 69–80.

11. Witzig TE, Gordon LI, Cabanillas F, *et al.* (2002). Randomized controlled trial of yttrium-90-labeled ibritumomab tiuxetan radioimmunotherapy versus rituximab immunotherapy for patients with relapsed or refractory low-grade, follicular, or transformed B-cell non-Hodgkin's lymphoma. *Journal of Clinical Oncology* **20**(10): 2453–63.

12. Davis TA, Kaminski MS, Leonard JP, *et al.* (2004). The radioisotope contributes significantly to the activity of radioimmunotherapy. *Clinical Cancer Research* **10**(23): 7792–8.

13. Press OW, Leonard JP, Coiffier B, Levy R, Timmerman J (2001). Immunotherapy of non-Hodgkin's lymphomas. *Hematology*, Am Soc Hematol Educ Program Vol. 1. 221–40.

14. Kaminski MS, Tuck M, Estes J, *et al.* (2005). 131I-tositumomab therapy as initial treatment for follicular lymphoma. *New England Journal of Medicine* **352**(5): 441–9.

15. Knox SJ, Meredith RF (2000). Clinical radioimmunotherapy. *Seminars in Radiation Oncology* **10**(2): 73–93.

16. Dyer MJ, Hale G, Hayhoe FG, Waldmann H (1989). Effects of CAMPATH-1 antibodies in vivo in patients with lymphoid malignancies: influence of antibody isotype. *Blood* **73**(6): 1431–9.

17. Goldenberg DM, Horowitz JA, Sharkey RM, *et al.* (1991). Targeting, dosimetry, and radioimmunotherapy of B-cell lymphomas with iodine-131-labeled LL2 monoclonal antibody. *Journal of Clinical Oncology* **9**(4): 548–64.

18. Hekman A, Honselaar A, Vuist WM, *et al.* (1991). Initial experience with treatment of human B cell lymphoma with anti-CD19 monoclonal antibody. *Cancer Immunology and Immunotherapy* **32**(6): 364–72.

19. Kaminski MS, Fig LM, Zasadny KR, *et al.* (1992). Imaging, dosimetry, and radioimmunotherapy with iodine 131-labeled anti-CD37 antibody in B-cell lymphoma. *Journal of Clinical Oncology* **10**(11): 1696–711.

20. Press OW, Eary JF, Appelbaum FR, *et al.* (1993). Radiolabeled-antibody therapy of B-cell lymphoma with autologous bone marrow support. *New England Journal of Medicine* **329**(17): 1219–24.

21. Brown RS, Kaminski MS, Fisher SJ, Chang AE, Wahl RL (1997). Intratumoral microdistribution of [131I]MB-1 in patients with B-cell lymphoma following radioimmunotherapy. *Nuclear Medicine and Biology* **24**(7): 657–63.

22. DeNardo GL, DeNardo SJ, Goldstein DS, *et al.* (1998). Maximum-tolerated dose, toxicity, and efficacy of (131)I-Lym-1 antibody for fractionated radioimmunotherapy of non-Hodgkin's lymphoma. *Journal of Clinical Oncology* **16**(10): 3246–56.

23. Kaminski MS, Zelenetz AD, Press OW, *et al.* (2001). Pivotal study of iodine I 131 tositumomab for chemotherapy-refractory low-grade or transformed low-grade B-cell non-Hodgkin's lymphomas. *Journal of Clinical Oncology* **19**(19): 3918–28.

24. Press OW (2003). Radioimmunotherapy for non-Hodgkin's lymphomas: a historical perspective. *Seminars in Oncology* **30**(2 Suppl. 4): 10–21.

25. Grossbard ML, Press OW, Appelbaum FR, Bernstein ID, Nadler LM (1992). Monoclonal antibody-based therapies of leukemia and lymphoma. *Blood* **80**(4): 863–78.

26. Shan D, Ledbetter JA, Press OW (1998). Apoptosis of malignant human B cells by ligation of CD20 with monoclonal antibodies. *Blood* **91**(5): 1644–52.

27. Shan D, Ledbetter JA, Press OW (2000). Signaling events involved in anti-CD20-induced apoptosis of malignant human B cells. *Cancer Immunology and Immunotherapy* **48**(12): 673–83.

28. Press OW, Rasey J (2000). Principles of radioimmunotherapy for hematologists and oncologists. *Seminars in Oncology* **27**(6 Suppl. 12): 62–73.

29. Goldenberg DM (2001). The role of radiolabeled antibodies in the treatment of non-Hodgkin's lymphoma: the coming of age of radioimmunotherapy. *Critical Reviews in Oncology/Hematology* **39**(1–2): 195–201.

30. Wagner HN, Jr, Wiseman GA, Marcus CS, *et al.* (2002). Administration guidelines for radioimmunotherapy of non-Hodgkin's lymphoma with (90)Y-labeled anti-CD20 monoclonal antibody. *Journal of Nuclear Medicine* **43**(2): 267–72.

31. Wahl RL (2005). Tositumomab and (131)I therapy in non-Hodgkin's lymphoma. *Journal of Nuclear Medicine* **46** (Suppl. 1): 128–40S.

32. Vriesendorp HM, Quadri SM, Stinson RL, *et al.* (1992). Selection of reagents for human radioimmunotherapy. *International Journal of Radiation Oncology, Biology, Physics* **22**: 37–45.

33. DeNardo GL, O'Donnell RT, Shen S, *et al.* (2001). Radiation dosimetry for 90Y-2IT-BAD-Lym-1 extrapolated from pharmacokinetics using 111In-2IT-BAD-Lym-1 in patients with non-Hodgkin's lymphoma. *Journal of Nuclear Medicine* **41**(5): 952–8.

34. Sharkey RM, Behr TM, Mattes MJ, *et al.* (1997). Advantage of residualizing radiolabels for an internalizing antibody against the B-cell lymphoma antigen, CD22. *Cancer Immunology and Immunotherapy* **44**(3): 179–88.

35. Press OW, Shan D, Howell-Clark J, *et al.* (1996). Comparative metabolism and retention of iodine-125, yttrium-90, and indium-111 radioimmunoconjugates by cancer cells. *Cancer Research* **56**(9): 2123–9.

36. DeNardo GL, Kukis DL, Shen S, DeNardo DA, Meares CF, Denardo SJ (1999). 67Cu-versus 131I-labeled Lym-1 antibody: comparative pharmacokinetics and dosimetry in patients with non-Hodgkin's lymphoma. *Clinical Cancer Research* **5**(3): 533–41.

37. McDevitt MR, Sgouros G, Finn RD, *et al.* (1998). Radioimmunotherapy with alpha-emitting nuclides. *European Journal of Nuclear Medicine* **25**(9): 1341–51.

38. Jurcic JG, Larson SM, Sgouros G, *et al.* (2002). Targeted alpha particle immunotherapy for myeloid leukemia. *Blood* **100**(4): 1233–9.

39. Zhang M, Yao Z, Garmestani K, *et al.* (2002). Pretargeting radioimmunotherapy of a murine model of adult T-cell leukemia with the alpha-emitting radionuclide, bismuth 213. *Blood* **100**: 208–16.

40. Zhang M, Zhang Z, Garmestani K, *et al.* (2003). Pretarget radiotherapy with an anti-CD25 antibody-streptavidin fusion protein was effective in therapy of leukemia/lymphoma xenografts. *Proceedings of the National Academy of Sciences USA* **100**(4): 1891–5.

41. Oh P, Li Y, Yu J, *et al.* (2004). Subtractive proteomic mapping of the endothelial surface in lung and solid tumours for tissue-specific therapy. *Nature* **429**(6992): 629–35.

42. Wahl RL (2003). The clinical importance of dosimetry in radioimmunotherapy with tositumomab and iodine I 131 tositumomab. *Seminars in Oncology* **30**(2 Suppl. 4): 31–8.

43. Kaminski MS, Zasadny KR, Francis IR, *et al.* (1993). Radioimmunotherapy of B-cell lymphoma with [131I]anti-B1 (anti-CD20) antibody. *New England Journal of Medicine* **329**(7): 459–65.

44. Witzig TE, White CA, Wiseman GA, *et al.* (1999). Phase I/II trial of IDEC-Y2B8 radioimmunotherapy for treatment of relapsed or refractory CD20(+) B-cell non-Hodgkin's lymphoma. *Journal of Clinical Oncology* **17**(12): 3793–803.

45. Wiseman GA, Kornmehl E, Leigh B, *et al.* (2003). Radiation dosimetry results and safety correlations from 90Y-ibritumomab tiuxetan radioimmunotherapy for relapsed or refractory non-Hodgkin's lymphoma: combined data from 4 clinical trials. *Journal of Nuclear Medicine* **44**(3): 465–74.

46. Witzig TE, White CA, Gordon LI, *et al.* (2003). Safety of yttrium-90 ibritumomab tiuxetan radioimmunotherapy for relapsed low-grade, follicular, or transformed non-Hodgkin's lymphoma. *Journal of Clinical Oncology* **21**(7): 1263–70.

47. Illidge T, Bayne M, Zivanovic M, Du Y, Lewingtan V, Johnson P (2004). Phase I/II study of fractionated radioimmunotherapy in relapsed low grade non-Hodgkin's lymphoma. *Blood* **104**(11): 131.

48. Fisher DR (2000). Internal dosimetry for systemic radiation therapy. *Seminars in Radiation Oncology* **10**(2): 123–32.

49. Wiseman GA, Leigh B, Erwin WD, *et al.* (2002). Radiation dosimetry results for Zevalin radioimmunotherapy of rituximab-refractory non-Hodgkin lymphoma. *Cancer* **94**(4 Suppl.): 1349–57.

50. Dewaraja YK, Wilderman SJ, Ljungberg M, Koral KF, Zasadny K, Kaminiski MS (2005). Accurate dosimetry in 131I radionuclide therapy using patient-specific, 3-dimensional methods for SPECT reconstruction and absorbed dose calculation. *Journal of Nuclear Medicine* **46**(5): 840–9.

51. Wiseman GA, White CA, Witzig TE, *et al.* (1999). Radioimmunotherapy of relapsed non-Hodgkin's lymphoma with zevalin, a 90Y-labeled anti-CD20 monoclonal antibody. *Clinical Cancer Research* **5**(10 Suppl.): 3281–6s.

52. Schilder R, Molina A, Bartlett N, *et al.* (2004). Follow-up results of a phase II study of ibritumomab tiuxetan radioimmunotherapy in patients with relapsed or refractory low-grade, follicular, or transformed B-cell non-Hodgkin's lymphoma and mild thrombocytopenia. *Cancer Biotherapy and Radiopharmaceutics* **19**(4): 478–81.

53. Hohenstein MA, Augustine SC, Rutar F, Vose JM (2003). Establishing an institutional model for the administration of tositumomab and iodine I 131 tositumomab. *Seminars in Oncology* **30**(2 Suppl. 4): 39–49.

54. Gordon LI, Witzig TE, Wiseman GA, *et al.* (2002). Yttrium 90 ibritumomab tiuxetan radioimmunotherapy for relapsed or refractory low-grade non-Hodgkin's lymphoma. *Seminars in Oncology* **29**(1 Suppl. 2): 87–92.

55. Czuczman M (2002). Zevalin radioimmunotherapy is not associated with an increased incidence of secondary myelodysplastic syndrome (MDS) or acute myelogenous leukemia (AML). *Blood* **100**: 375a.

56. Wiseman G, Leigh B, Witzig T, Gomseb D, White C (2001). Radiation exposure is very low to the family members of patients treated with yttrium-90 Zevalin anti-CD20 monoclonal antibody therapy for lymphoma. *European Journal of Nuclear Medicine* **28**(8): 1198 (Abstract PS479).

57. Wiseman GA, White CA, Sparks RB, *et al.* (2001). Biodistribution and dosimetry results from a phase III prospectively randomized controlled trial of Zevalin radioimmunotherapy for low-grade, follicular, or transformed B-cell non-Hodgkin's lymphoma. *Critical Reviews in Oncology/Hematology* **39**(1–2): 181–94.

58. Zelenetz AD (2003). A clinical and scientific overview of tositumomab and iodine I 131 tositumomab. *Seminars in Oncology* **30**(2 Suppl. 4): 22–30.

59. Liu SY, Eary JF, Petersdorf SH, *et al.* (1998). Follow-up of relapsed B-cell lymphoma patients treated with iodine-131-labeled anti-CD20 antibody and autologous stem-cell rescue. *Journal of Clinical Oncology* **16**(10): 3270–8.

60. DeNardo GL, Mirick GR, Kroger LA, Bradt BM, Lamborn KR, DeNardo SJ (2003). Characterization of human IgG antimouse antibody in patients with B-cell malignancies. *Clinical Cancer Research* **9**(10 Pt 2): 4013–21S.

61. Bennett JM, Kaminski MS, Leonard JP, *et al.* (2005). Assessment of treatment-related myelodysplastic syndromes and acute myeloid leukemia in patients with non-Hodgkin lymphoma treated with tositumomab and iodine I131 tositumomab. *Blood* **105**(12): 4576–82.

62. Wilder RB, DeNardo GL, DeNardo SJ (1996). Radioimmunotherapy: recent results and future directions. *Journal of Clinical Oncology* **14**(4): 1383–400.

63. Sharkey RM, Goldenberg DM (2005). Perspectives on cancer therapy with radiolabeled monoclonal antibodies. *Journal of Nuclear Medicine* **46** (Suppl. 1): 115–27S.

64. DeNardo GL, DeNardo SJ, O'Grady LF, Levy NB, Adams GP, Mills SL (1990). Fractionated radioimmunotherapy of B-cell malignancies with 131I-Lym-1. *Cancer Research* **50**(3 Suppl.): 1014–6s.

65. DeNardo GL, DeNardo SJ, Lamborn KR, *et al.* (1998). Low-dose, fractionated radioimmunotherapy for B-cell malignancies using 131I-Lym-1 antibody. *Cancer Biotherapy and Radiopharmaceutics* **13**(4): 239–54.

66. Juweid ME, Stadtmauer E, Hajjar G, *et al.* (1999). Pharmacokinetics, dosimetry, and initial therapeutic results with 131I- and (111)In-/90Y-labeled humanized LL2 anti-CD22 monoclonal antibody in patients with relapsed, refractory non-Hodgkin's lymphoma. *Clinical Cancer Research* **5**(10 Suppl.): 3292–303s.

67. Hajjar G, Sharkey R, Barton J *et al.* (2001). Interim results of a phase I/II radioimmunotherapy trial in relapsed/refractory non-Hodgkin's lymphoma (NHL) patients given Y-90 labeled anti-CD22 humanised monoclonal antibodies. *Blood* **98**(11 Pt 1): 611a (Abstract 2560).

68. Kaminski MS, Zasadny KR, Francis IR, *et al.* (1996). Iodine-131-anti-B1 radioimmunotherapy for B-cell lymphoma. *Journal of Clinical Oncology* **14**(7): 1974–81.

69. Friedberg JW, Fisher RI (2004). Iodine-131 tositumomab (Bexxar(R)): radioimmunoconjugate therapy for indolent and transformed B-cell non-Hodgkin's lymphoma. *Expert Review of Anticancer Therapy* **4**: 18–26.

70. Kaminiski MS, Zelenetz A, Leonard J, Saleh M, Jain V (2002). Bexxar radioimmunotherapy produces a substantial number of durable complete responses in patients with multiply relapsed or refractory low grade or transformed low grade non-Hodgkin's lymphoma. *Blood* **100**(11 Pt 1): 356a (Abstract 1382).

71. Gregory S, Kaminiski MS, Zelenetz A, Jain V (2002). Characteristics of patients with replased and refractory low grade non-Hodgkin's lymphoma who sustained durable responses following treatment with tositumomab and iodine-131 tositumomab (Bexxar). *Blood* **100**(11 Pt 2): 312b (Abstract 4791).

72. Horning S, Younes A, Lucas J, Podoloff DA, Jain V (2002). Rituximab treatment failures: Tositumomab and iodine-131 tositumomab (Bexxar) can produce meaningful durable responses. *Blood* **100**(11 Pt 1): 357a (Abstract 1385).

73. Coleman M, Kaminiski MS, Knox SJ, Zelenetz A, Vose J (2003). The BEXXAR therapeutic regimen (Tositumomab and Iodine I 131 Tositumomab) produced durable complete remissions in heavily pretreated patients with non-Hodgkins lymphoma (NHL), rituximab-relapsed/refractory disease, and rituximab-naive disease. *Blood* **102**(11): 29a (Abstract 89).

74. Koral KF, Dewaraja Y, Li J, *et al.* (2003). Update on hybrid conjugate-view SPECT tumor dosimetry and response in 131I-tositumomab therapy of previously untreated lymphoma patients. *Journal of Nuclear Medicine* **44**(3): 457–64.

75. Gordon LI, Molina A, Witzig T, *et al.* (2004). Durable responses after ibritumomab tiuxetan radioimmunotherapy for CD20+ B-cell lymphoma: long-term follow-up of a phase 1/2 study. *Blood* **103**(12): 4429–31.

76. Gordon LI, Witzig T, Molina A, *et al.* (2004). Yttrium 90-labeled ibritumomab tiuxetan radioimmunotherapy produces high response rates and durable remissions in patients with previously treated B-cell lymphoma. *Clinical Lymphoma* **5**(2): 98–101.

77. Morschhauser F, Huglo D, Martinelli G, *et al.* (2004). Yttrium-90 ibritumomab tiuxetan (Zevalin) for patients with replased/refractory diffuse large B-cell lymphoma not appropriate for autologous stem cell transplantation: Results of an open-label phase II trial. *Blood* **104**(11): 41a (Abstract 130).

78. Zelenetz AD (1999). Radioimmunotherapy for lymphoma. *Current Opinion in Oncology* **11**(5): 375–80.

79. Illidge TM, Johnson PW (2000). The emerging role of radioimmunotherapy in haematological malignancies. *British Journal of Haematology* **108**(4): 679–88.

80. Koral KF, Kaminski MS, Wahl RL (2003). Correlation of tumor radiation-absorbed dose with response is easier to find in previously untreated patients. *Journal of Nuclear Medicine* **44**(9): 1541–3.

81. Britton KE (2004). Radioimmunotherapy of non-Hodgkin's lymphoma. *Journal of Nuclear Medicine* **45**(5): 924–5.

82. Postema EJ (2004). Dosimetry and radioimmunotherapy of non-Hodgkin's lymphoma. *Journal of Nuclear Medicine* **45**(12): 2126–7.

83. Goldenberg DM, Sharkey RM (2005). Radioimmunotherapy of non-Hodgkin's lymphoma revisited. *Journal of Nuclear Medicine* **46**(2): 383–4.

84. Cragg MS, French RR, Glennie MJ (1999). Signaling antibodies in cancer therapy. *Current Opinion in Immunology* **11**(5): 541–7.

85. Cragg MS, Glennie MJ (2004). Antibody specificity controls in vivo effector mechanisms of anti-CD20 reagents. *Blood* **103**(7): 2738–43.

86. Bannerji R, Kitada S, Flinn IW, *et al.* (2003). Apoptotic-regulatory and complement-protecting protein expression in chronic lymphocytic leukemia: relationship to in vivo rituximab resistance. *Journal of Clinical Oncology* **21**(8): 1466–71.

87. Chan HT, Hughes D, French RR, *et al.* (2003). CD20-induced lymphoma cell death is independent of both caspases and its redistribution into triton X-100 insoluble membrane rafts. *Cancer Research* **63**(17): 5480–9.

88. Illidge TM, Cragg MS, McBride HM, French RR, Glennie MJ (1999). The importance of antibody-specificity in determining successful radioimmunotherapy of B-cell lymphoma. *Blood* **94**: 233–43.

89. Du Y, Honeychurch J, Bayne M, *et al.* (2004). Antibody-induced intracellular signaling works in combination with radiation to eradicate lymphoma in radioimmunotherapy. *Blood* **103**(4): 1485–94.

Chapter 8

Other therapeutic uses of radioisotopes

Peter Hoskin

8.1 Introduction

Radionuclides may be used for proliferative haematological disorders, the most common of which is polycythaemia rubra vera and primary thrombocytosis. Radioisotopes in liquid or colloid form can in principle be administered to any body cavity and thereby, using short range decay products, deliver radiation doses to cavity surfaces. This property has been exploited in a number of scenarios. These include potential treatments for pleural effusion, ascites, and pericardial effusion. They have also been employed for the treatment of synovitis associated with rheumatoid arthritis and haemophilia.

8.2 Radionuclide therapy in haematology

The common isotope use for haematological disorders is phosphorus (^{32}P). ^{32}P as discussed in Chapter 1 is a pure β emitter with maximum energy 1.71 MeV having a mean range in tissue of 3 mm and maximum range of 8 mm. Its half-life is 14.3 days. It is selectively taken up into bone marrow, spleen, and liver. It is incorporated in the calcium phosphate of the bone lying adjacent to the endosteum and also the active bone marrow cells. Approximately 30% of an injected dose is absorbed in mineral bone. The biological half-life in marrow is 7–9 days and the absorbed dose to bone marrow is approximately 6.5 mGy per MBq administered, although there is considerable variation[1,2].

8.3 Polycythaemia

Polycythaemia vera is the commonest use of ^{32}P. Its relative efficacy alongside other agents including regular venesection and alkylating drugs such as chlorambucil, busulfan, and hydroxyurea remains uncertain. One randomized trial by the Polycythaemia Vera Study Group compared in 431 patients ^{32}P with chlorambucil and phlebotomy. The chlorambucil arm of the study was discontinued early because of an excess of secondary acute leukaemia[3]. The results of ^{32}P were highly favourable with a median survival of 13–16 years from onset of the disease approaching a normal life expectancy for patients with this condition. In standard doses there are few complications and no significant myelosuppression was seen. It is associated with a lower incidence of thrombotic and haemorrhagic complications compared with phlebotomy and gives a similar response rate to hydroxyurea[4].

The dose scheduling used in this study was an induction dose of 2.3 mCi/m^2 intravenously, the maximum dose not exceeding 5 mCi. A second dose was repeated 12 weeks later if the patient still required phlebotomy or had less than a 25% decrement in platelet or white cell count. ^{32}P was contraindicated where the platelet count was less than $100,000 \times 10^9$/l or the total white count less than 3000×10^9/l.

There is an increased risk of transformation in polycythaemia to myelodysplasia and acute leukaemia. The role of ^{32}P in this is uncertain.

8.4 Essential thrombocythaemia

Essential thrombocythaemia is also treated readily with ^{32}P. The Polycythaemia Vera Study Group has again investigated this with a randomized trial comparing ^{32}P with melphalan demonstrating equivalent complete remission rates[5] but a relatively high incidence of acute leukaemia seen in 30% of a subgroup of that study. The subgroups, however, are small and it is not possible to conclude that this was greater in the patients receiving ^{32}P than alkylating agent or hydroxyurea. It was seen in five of seven patients given hydroxyurea initially who later received ^{32}P[6].

Current recommendations are for ^{32}P to be considered in polycythaemia and thrombocythaemia in patients over the age of 70 while in younger patients hydroxyurea may be a more appropriate treatment, although this depends upon the absolute risk of leukaemia.

8.5 Leukaemias

The use of ^{32}P in chronic myeloid and lymphocytic leukaemias is now essentially of historic interest. The management of chronic myeloid leukaemia has been overtaken by advances in chemotherapy and particularly the development of imatinib methysylate (Glivec).

In chronic lymphocytic leukaemia there are data from small series that suggest this treatment was effective in reducing high lymphocyte counts and maintaining them within a range of 30×10^9/l or less. Prior to the use of alkylating agents and more modern combination therapies it was thought that ^{32}P resulted in an increase in life expectancy over supportive treatment alone by a year or so. There is no proven role for ^{32}P in chronic lymphocytic leukaemia today.

8.6 Intracavitary radionuclide therapy

A potential body cavity such as the peritoneal cavity or pleural cavity when distended with fluid is an ideal opportunity for the installation of a radionuclide. Radioisotopes in colloid solutions have been used for both pleural effusions and ascites. They are a rational approach to the treatment of malignant effusions, in principle delivering a dose of low penetration radiation to the entire membrane surface from which the effusion is being produced and the fluid within the cavity, thus targeting the malignant cells both on the membrane surface and floating free in the fluid.

Both colloidal gold (^{198}Au) and colloidal chromic phosphate (^{32}P) have been used. ^{32}P has greater β energy penetration than gold, which also has a shorter half-life. There is also 5% of γ emission from gold, which has a potential disadvantage, although it does enable the distribution of the isotope to be seen using a gamma camera. When ^{32}P is used a tracer dose of technetium may be given if imaging is required. In general, therefore, radioactive phosphorous colloidal solution has been chosen in preference to colloidal gold.

Estimates of dose distribution using gold or phosphorus with technetium have demonstrated that often there is uneven distribution of the radioisotope within the cavity and this is a potential disadvantage. This is particularly the case in the abdomen, which is a larger more complex cavity and may be compounded by the effects of previous surgical interference.

There are limited data on the efficacy of treatment by this route. Small case series suggest that about 50% of patients may benefit by having control of the effusion with no further re-accumulation. Toxicity is negligible[7,8].

Colloidal chromic phosphate has been used in pericardial effusions with a reported response rate of 71%[7].

Intracavitary radioisotope therapy is not commonly used today. It is complex to deliver requiring careful installation with a risk of isotope spillage from intrapleural or intraperitoneal catheters. There are concerns with regard to achieving uniform dosimetry, although the need for this to achieve control of an effusion has been questioned. These factors together with the increasing availability of effective systemic chemotherapy has reduced the use of radionuclides for the control of effusions. It is perhaps an underused potentially effective treatment modality in this setting.

8.7 **Radiosynovectomy**

Synovitis is a prominent feature of rheumatoid arthritis and is also a feature in haemophilia where a chronic hypertrophic synovitis occurs secondary to recurrent haemarthroses. Formal surgical synovectomy is one option but radionuclide synovectomy can be undertaken as an alternative. Intra-articular colloidal gold (^{198}Au) or yttrium-silicate (^{90}Y) have been used. Colloidal gold has a particle size of 5–10 nm with a maximum penetration in the synovium of 3.6 mm. Colloid yttrium-silicate has a particle size of about 100 nm, is a pure β emitter with maximal energy 2.2 MeV penetrating to a depth of 11 mm in the synovium. Both have a physical half-life of 2.7 days. More recent studies have also used colloidal chromic phosphate (^{32}P)[9].

Administration is simple injection of the colloidal solution into the intra-articular space, which is usually well tolerated. There are a small number of case series reporting the efficacy. Postinjection a flare of synovitis is seen in 5–15% of patients. Response criteria in this setting are not uniformly defined. Overall, 50–60% of patients are reported to have a good result with control of pain and improved mobility and a further 25–30% a lesser improvement[9,10]. In haemophilia a mid- and long-term efficacy of 75–80% is reported[11]. An additional benefit of radionuclide treatment in this setting is to cause sclerosis and reduced vascularization of the synovium and hence a reduction in the incidence of haemarthrosis. Repeat treatments in 20–25% of patients are described. Systemic side-effects are not expected and other than a transient flare of local symptoms major complications in the joint are not reported. Comparative non-randomized data against surgical synovectomy suggests the results at 1 and 2 years are equivalent. Longer-term benefits are not well evaluated. In practice this approach is not widespread.

References

1. Berlin NI (2000). Treatment of the myeloproliferative disorders with ^{32}P. *European Journal of Haematology* **65**: 1–7.

2. Roberts BE, Smith AH (1997). Use of radioactive phosphorus in haematology. *Blood Reviews* **11**: 146–53.

3. Berk PD, Goldberg JD, Silverstein MN, *et al.* (1981). Increased incidence of acute leukaemia in polycythemia vera associated with chlorambucil therapy. *New England Journal of Medicine* **304**: 441–7.

4. Berk PD, Goldberg JD, Donovan P, Fruchtman SM, Berlinn NI, Wasserman LR (1986). Therapeutic recommendations in polycythemia vera based on Polycythemia Vera Study Group Protocols. *Seminars in Hematology* **23**: 132–43.

5. Murphy S, Rosenthal D, Wenfeld A *et al.* (1982). Essential thrombocythemia: response during first year of therapy with melphalan and radioactive phosphorus: a Polycythemia Vera Study Group Report. *Cancer Chemotherapy Reports* **66**: 1495–500.

6. Murphy S, Peterson P, Iland HJ, Laslo J (1997). Experience of the Polycythemia Vera Study Group with essential thrombocythemia: a final report on diagnostic criteria, survival and leukaemic transition by treatment. *Seminars in Hematology* **34**: 29–39.

7. Croll M, Brady LW (1979). Intracavitary uses of colloids. *Seminars in Nuclear Medicine* **9**: 108–13.

8. Mohlen KH, Beller FK (1979). Use of radioactive gold in the treatment of pleural effusions caused by metastatic cancer. *Cancer Research and Clinical Oncology* **94**: 81–5.

9. Lee P (1982). The efficacy and safety of radiosynovectomy. *Journal of Rheumatology* **9**: 165–168.

10. Boerbooms AM, Buijs CAM, Danen M, van de Putte LBA, Vandenbroucke JP (1985). Radio-synovectomy in chronic synovitis of the knee joints in patients with rheumatoid arthritis. *European Journal of Nuclear Medicine* **10**: 446–9.

11. Rodriguz-Merchan EC (2003). Radionuclide synovectomy (Radiosynoviorthesis) in hemophilia: a very efficient and single procedure. *Seminars in Thrombosis and Hemostasis* **29**: 97–100.

Chapter 9

Radioprotection and regulatory aspects of radioisotope therapy

Stephen Evans, Brenda Pratt

9.1 European Directives and UK legislation

Health and safety legislation in the UK is developed from European Directives produced by the European Community. Much of the legislation governing the medical uses of ionizing radiations arises from the Basic Safety Standard (BSS) Directive (96/29/Euratom) published in 1996[1] and the Medical Exposure (ME) Directive (97/43/Euratom) published in 1997[2]. Both directives had to be implemented by member states into their country's legislation by the year 2000.

The BSS directive was largely implemented in the UK by the Health and Safety Executive (HSE) in regulations entitled The Ionising Radiations Regulations 1999 (IRR99)[3]. These regulations are supported by an HSE Approved Code of Practice and Guidance[4]. The ME directive was implemented in the UK by the Department of Health (DH) in the Ionising Radiation (Medical Exposure) Regulations 2000 (IR(ME)R)[5]. Further guidance on the implementation of these regulations is provided in the Medical and Dental Guidance Notes[6].

9.2 Controlling doses to staff and members of the public

IRR99 sets out the way in which employers (referred to in these regulations as radiation employers) must comply with the use of ionizing radiations in their workplace. These regulations set down dose limits for occupational exposure, identify the need to designate areas as controlled or supervised radiation areas with local rules to be followed by anyone entering such areas. To ensure compliance with the regulations, a radiation employer has to appoint a radiation protection adviser (RPA) who must hold a certificate of competence to act as an RPA. Radiation protection supervisors (RPSs) must also be appointed (normally staff working in the department or ward) to ensure staff comply with the local rules for their area. Names of the appointed RPSs must be written into their local rules. The following sections will detail some of the relevant matters for work involving unsealed source therapies.

9.2.1 Annual dose limits

All persons, excepting patients and comforters and carers (see later), are only allowed, by law, to be exposed to ionizing radiation in the workplace up to certain dose limits. The levels at which these limits are set for occupational whole body exposures are designed to be proportionate to roughly the median level of risks that are found in other industries. The dose limits for extremities and lens of eye are set such that the deterministic dose threshold levels for effects such as skin erythema and cataract formation would never be reached. The level of risk for members of the public are kept to a level that is commensurate with typical natural background radiation levels that result from exposure to cosmic rays and from the earth itself due to its radioactive nature (ignoring exposure to radon gas, which is highly variable).

Table 9.1 lists the annual effective dose limits under IRR99. The effective dose provides a dose value that equates to the same radiation risk to the person if the exposure had been uniform over the whole body. This is calculated by summing up the equivalent doses (see below) to different organs after weighting each of these exposures by the normalized radiosensitivities of the different organs throughout the body. To derive the excess lifetime fatal cancer risk from any exposure to ionizing radiation the effective dose in Sieverts (Sv) could be multiplied by 0.05. Alternatively the risk could be thought of as 1 in 20 000 per mSv, so, for example, an effective dose of 2 mSv would result in a 1 in 10 000 excess lifetime fatal cancer risk. Both these values are rough approximations for an average 40 year old in normal health.

Also in Table 9.1 is shown the equivalent dose limits to organs and tissues under IRR99. The equivalent dose is the absorbed dose to the organ or tissue

Table 9.1 Annual dose limits

	Employees	Public and all persons under 16 years
Effective dose (mSv)	20	1
Equivalent doses (mSv):		
Lens of eye	150	15
Skin*	500	50
Hands, forearms, feet, ankles	500	50

*Skin dose averaged over 1 cm^2 of skin.

multiplied by a radiation weighting factor that relates to the radiobiological effectiveness of the type of radiation involved. For photons and βs the radiation weighting factor is 1 and for αs the factor is 20.

Staff must be designated as classified persons if their annual dose exceeds 3/10ths of any dose limit. To ensure compliance with this requirement, employers should designate a person as classified if their dose is likely to approach 3/10ths of any one of these limits. To enable a person to become designated as a classified person they must first undergo a baseline medical examination by an HSE-appointed doctor to ensure there are no underlying medical conditions that would prohibit their designation. Once declared fit for this designation, they must be monitored by a personal dosimetry service that has been approved by the HSE and their annual dose records will be sent to the Central Index of Dose Information maintained by the Radiation Division of the Health Protection Agency (HPA-RD) (formally the NRPB). Annually thereafter the classified person must be seen by an appointed doctor who will make a statement that they are fit to continue being classified.

In some industries the employer may decide to designate all radiation workers as classified persons regardless of the dose they are likely to receive. These employers may see some benefit in having all their staff undergo an annual medical and feel more secure should any of their staff receive a dose above 3/10ths of any dose limit.

In the National Health Service (NHS) in England and Wales, it is uncommon for staff to be designated. Here employers and employees may see some benefit in not classifying persons so ensuring doses staff receive are kept below the level for designations. In this latter case, it is still commonplace for staff to be monitored by an approved dosimetry service.

9.2.2 Design of facilities

Some treatments can be given on an outpatient basis and the most common therapy is radioiodine for the treatment of hyperthyroidism. Radioiodine is administered orally either in liquid or dry powder capsule form. Other treatments using β emitters, ^{32}P and ^{89}Sr are administered intravenously. These are usually administered in the nuclear medicine department.

Therapies involving large activities (GBq level) of radionuclides will require the patient to be admitted to hospital. Patients undergoing unsealed source therapies should ideally be admitted to purpose-built units with en-suite facilities. A radioisotope suite requires a separate but connected support area in the same location as the treatment rooms. The support area must have sufficient space to contain contaminated linen and possibly waste, monitoring instruments, washing machine, and tumble dryer. A typical layout

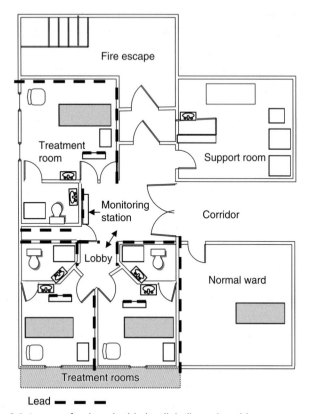

Fig. 9.1 Layout of a three-bedded radioiodine suite with support room.

of a three-bedded radioisotope suite is shown in Fig. 9.1. All rooms should be decorated so that they are easy to decontaminate. Floors should be of continuous sealed vinyl with lipped wall edges and walls should have smooth sealed surfaces. Items of furniture should, where practicable, be made of non-porous (e.g. vinyl) materials, which are able to be wipe cleaned. Shower cubicles should be easy to wipe clean with shower doors used in preference to shower curtains. It is also worth considering installing radiation monitoring equipment in a fixed position in the room to enable serial measurements to be made of the patient's radionuclide retention. This eliminates the need for staff to enter the treatment room to obtain these measurements and thus reduce staff exposure.

In siting the suite, consideration should be given to the possible dose rates in the surrounding areas, particularly those with public access. Significant shielding will be required for walls, floor, and ceiling areas. If shielding has not been established during the initial building phase (e.g. a new suite is designed within an existing establishment) consideration must be given to the possible need for significant additional lead shielding. For example, if a suite was to be located in a room with partition walls and hollow block floors and ceiling, it might be necessary to add 10 mm or more thick lead slabs to the walls, floor, and ceiling. If drainage from the suite passes through areas of high occupancy the drain pipe may need to be shielded. The RPA or suitably qualified medical physicist should be contacted to provide assistance with the extra shielding requirements.

9.2.3 Controlled areas

Areas or rooms where radiation is used or is present (e.g. a patient may have been administered with a radiopharmaceutical) must be designated as controlled radiation areas if there is a likelihood for staff to receive either a significant exposure (e.g. the external dose rate is more than 7.5 µSv/h averaged over the working day) or an external exposure that could result in a dose of more than 3/10th of a relevant dose limit. Similarly, an area must be designated as a controlled area if there is a likelihood of contamination being spread outside the area. The RPS (see Section 9.2.5) will ensure that staff entering these areas comply with the written local rules for the areas. Non-classified staff are only allowed entry to these areas under written arrangements that will stipulate the particular conditions of entry. For example, staff must read the local rules and be authorized by the RPS to enter the area. It should be noted that where a room has been designated as a classified area because there is the potential for contamination, each time a member of staff leaves the room it will be necessary for them to monitor their hands and feet and a record of the monitoring will need to be maintained. Hand and feet monitoring stations with automatic recording might be an advantage in such areas. For example, these monitors may be placed at the exit to a radioiodine therapy suite.

9.2.4 Supervised areas

Areas that do not require special procedures to restrict significant exposures nor give rise to a spread of contamination need not be designated as controlled areas. However, if a person is likely to receive an effective dose of more than 1 mSv in a year (or 1/10th of any relevant dose limit), or if it is necessary to keep the conditions of the area under review, it should be designated as a supervised area. An example of such an area could be the support room of a treatment suite where waste from the patients who have been administered with a radionuclide is present. In normal circumstances, there would not be a likelihood of significant spread of contamination. It might also be necessary to designate an area immediately outside a therapy room as a supervised area to restrict the occupancy at the exit to the room due to the potential for high external dose rates. However, if it is reasonably foreseeable that a patient may become incontinent or sick, the area may need to become temporarily changed to a controlled area. Classification as a supervised area may be more desirable than designation as a controlled area, as it would otherwise be necessary for staff to monitor themselves (hand and feet) each time they exit the area which may be impractical.

Designation of the radioisotope suite

Access to a controlled area should be prohibited to persons unconnected with the work of the area unless they can follow specific instructions. The external dose rates at the unshielded entrance (e.g. door open or not shielded) to the treatment room can be high when the patient is near to the door, which might result in the need for the area to be designated as a controlled or supervised area (see above section). Rooms with shielded maze entrances may not require their entrances to become designated areas. Ideally, all treatment rooms and the support room should be within a self-contained suite with a lobby area off which the rooms are situated. The entrance to the suite can either be designated as a supervised area with the treatment rooms designated as separate controlled areas, or, alternatively, the entrance to the suite (and thereby the whole of the suite) could be designated as a controlled area. Both options have advantages and disadvantages. In the former case, a member of staff may enter the lobby and support rooms that have been designated as supervised areas and would not need to monitor themselves when they exit the suite (as they have not entered a controlled area). However, each time staff leave any one of the treatment rooms they should monitor their hands and feet. In the latter case, staff only need to monitor their hands and feet when they leave the suite. However, they would need to monitor themselves each time they exit the suite even if they had only entered the lobby area (as it is controlled). It must be noted that records of monitoring need to be maintained to demonstrate compliance with this requirement. The option decided upon should result from a prior risk assessment. Once an area has been designated as a controlled area it must have a placard with an appropriate warning sign that identifies it as a controlled area with the radiation trefoil and a notice that the access is restricted to authorized persons. Pictograms and supplementary text should also be present to provide sufficient information alerting employees to the types of hazards present (e.g. risks from external radiation and contamination).

9.2.5 **Local rules and radiation protection supervisors**

Staff who enter any designated radiation area must comply with local rules that identify the key instructions to restrict exposure in the area. Other persons (e.g. service engineers or visitors) require specific authorization to enter a controlled area to ensure the key elements with the local rules to restrict exposure are maintained.

The employer is responsible for ensuring these local rules are in place and must appoint a suitable and appropriately trained employee as a radiation protection supervisor (RPS) to secure compliance with the local rules. The suitability of the appointment of the RPS should be made in consultation with the RPA. The employer should make the duties of the RPS clear in writing. Once the appointment is made, the name of the RPS should be listed in the local rules. It is also good practice to display the name of the RPS on the door notice boards. It is useful for the RPS to keep a list of all staff that they have authorized to enter the controlled areas under their supervision. The RPS should be satisfied that these staff have demonstrated they are able to follow the procedures identified in the local rules to restrict their exposure.

9.2.6 **Monitoring**

Staff entering controlled areas will require some form of dose assessment. In the case of non-classified staff this monitoring is required to demonstrate the doses received are below 3/10th of any relevant dose limit. Whole body dose assessments are most usually accomplished using film badges or thermoluminescent dosimeters worn at waist or chest level. In addition, staff administering the radionuclide as well as those dispensing radiopharmaceuticals will also require finger dose measurements normally by means of thermoluminescent dosimeter chips contained within plastic finger rings or stalls.

Monitoring of hands, clothing, and any area where unsealed radioactive sources have been used, using either a Geiger counter or scintillation monitor, should be a matter of routine to check for contamination. Calibrated (within the last 12 months) contamination monitors must be readily available for such monitoring and appropriate records of the monitoring must be maintained.

9.2.7 **Practical controls**

Patients should be encouraged to be as self-caring as possible to keep staff doses low. If it is necessary for staff to enter the treatment room good working practices must be adhered to that incorporate the three principal concepts of radiation protection: time, distance, and shielding. Time spent in close proximity to a radioactive patient or source should be kept to a minimum consistent with good practice. Similarly distance between staff and source should be maximized. All sources whether in vials or syringes should be appropriately shielded. Staff should wear plastic overshoes, aprons, and gloves. These must be discarded in designated bins when leaving the room. Mobile bed shields may also be necessary for staff working close to the patient. Access to the patient should be restricted to properly trained staff.

Advice and information should be available for staff who are exposed to radioactive patients on an occasional basis. A few basic guidelines should be set to ensure any exposure is kept as low as reasonably practicable (ALARP). For example, staff should be informed to wear protective clothing when dealing with bodily fluids and to avoid taking samples for other tests and schedule invasive procedures to avoid the period when the patient is radioactive.

Ideally the patient's visitors should not enter the room but be instructed to keep at the entrance to the patient's room. If this is not practicable and they need to enter the treatment room they must be given clear instructions on where they should sit and how long they may stay. In some circumstances they may also need to wear protective clothing. Visiting should normally be prohibited to pregnant women and children.

Additional preparation of the room can help to reduce contamination of surfaces. For example, Clingfilm (thin cellophane wraps) may be used to cover small items and handles and plastic sheets may be used to cover chairs. Male patients should be instructed to sit on the toilet and it might help during decontamination of the room if an absorbent disposable mat (e.g. Benchcote) is taped to the floor at the toilet area and any other areas where contamination is likely.

Crockery and cutlery used by the patient should either be disposable or there should be a system in place to wash items from these treatment rooms separately from other ward items. Linen from the treatment rooms should be monitored and if contaminated, washed and/or stored before sent to the main hospital laundry. Waste from the room (e.g. newspapers, magazines, plastic water bottles, etc.) must also be monitored and if necessary stored to allow the radioactivity to decay before disposal.

After discharge of an in-patient, the room and contents must be monitored for contamination and if necessary, decontaminated with suitable detergents such as Decon. Moveable items that are not adequately decontaminated may be stored until the remaining activity has decayed. Non-removable contaminated items should be covered with plastic sheets and secured with radioactive warning tape.

9.2.8 Staff pregnancy and breast feeding

The dose limit to the abdomen of a female employee is 13 mSv in any consecutive 3-month period. The employer must ensure that females have been informed about the risks to the fetus and to inform the employer (preferably in writing) when they become pregnant or start breastfeeding. Once an employee informs the employer she is pregnant, the employer must ensure the fetus does not receive a radiation dose of more than 1 mSv throughout the remaining pregnancy. An individual risk assessment should be carried out for pregnant employees to determine whether their work would need to change. Pregnant employees should not be allowed to work in areas where there is a reasonable likelihood for internal contamination to occur or where the dose to the abdomen is likely to approach or exceed 1 mSv from external radiation.

Systems of work should ensure there would not be likelihood for significant internal contamination of staff involved in caring for patients being treated with unsealed radionuclides. In the small number of cases where a patient has been sick or incontinent, the likelihood that a member of staff would receive a significant amount of internal contamination should be low if standard safety measures are employed. In these circumstances there may be some benefit in carrying out sensitive whole body uptake measurements that would be likely to give reassurance to the employee.

Some hospitals may consider it inappropriate for pregnant staff to carry out decontamination procedures in order that the dose and risk to the fetus is zero. In some hospitals, where it is practicable, conservative measures may be taken once nursing staff have declared their pregnancy and they would not be expected to work in any controlled radiation area.

Staff involved in the preparation and administration of therapeutic levels of radioactive substances have the potential to receive a significant level of internal contamination (although the likelihood of this happening should be very low) and it may be prudent to restrict the activities of pregnant staff in these areas.

A radiological risk assessment of the work involved will provide the likelihood of a significant hazard to a fetus occurring. A generic assessment would not, however, address the level of anxiety and stress caused to the pregnant woman if she was working in an environment where there was a potential for her to be exposed or contaminated. For this reason alone, individual risk assessments are important, and different outcomes and solutions may apply to different individuals. In situations where the pregnant woman remains concerned about continuing to work with ionizing radiations after being carefully informed of the degree of hazard and likelihood of the hazard occurring, it would be appropriate for the employer to find alternate work for this employee.

Equally important, women who are breast feeding should not work in areas where internal or external contamination (that could be transferred to an infant) is possible and similar guidance developed for pregnant women should be applied here. The employer should treat any woman returning from maternity leave as breast feeding unless or until otherwise informed.

9.2.9 Comforters and carers

Relatives and friends of patients being treated in hospital may be specially designated as comforters and carers if the exposure they receive has the potential to exceed the public dose limit. Persons who might become designated as comforter and carers must receive information on the risks associated with radiation exposures and be informed of the likely exposure they may receive in order that they can make an informed decision to become designated. They must also receive instruction and information to keep their dose as low as practicable. They are then able to consent to the exposure 'knowingly and willingly'. Dose limits for comforters and carers do not apply but it is good practice to restrict the dose to no more than 5 mSv per procedure. Here a procedure could be taken as the dose received by a comforter and carer from a course of treatments an individual patient undergoes during a year. The level at which this upper dose threshold is set represents the level likely to be received in a well managed operation and is referred to as a dose constraint. Comforters and carers should not normally be allowed to exceed the dose constraint unless exceptional circumstances prevail. It is advisable to provide some type of personal monitoring and keep records of the exposures. The typical information on risks and safety given to comforters and carer's is given in Appendix 9.1.

In general, pregnant women and children under 18 years of age (especially young children who are not normally considered to have the mental capacity to understand the risks and provide this consent) should not be allowed to act as comforters and carers. The dose to the fetus should be kept below 1 mSv and a dose constraint of 0.3 mSv would be appropriate. In special circumstances where a pregnant woman is likely to be involved in the care of a patient where the dose might exceed 1 mSv, informed consent may also need to be requested from the father of the unborn child who also has rights to the exposure of this fetus.

As stated previously, designation as a comforter and carer requires the person is exposed 'knowingly and willingly'. The annual dose other members of a household may receive from a patient returning home should be less than 1 mSv in a year as they are not 'knowingly and willingly' exposed. Ideally a dose constraint for these family members should be set at 0.3 mSv per procedure.

A good source of further information and guidance on comforters and carers is given in the report prepared for the HSE by the Royal Hallamshire hospital[7].

It should also be remembered that while in hospital, patients being treated with γ-emitting radionuclides (e.g. ^{131}I) are usually kept in shielded treatment rooms. Although the activity remaining in a patient will (normally) have decreased significantly before they are allowed to leave the hospital, family members may be exposed while sleeping in an adjacent room to the patient. It may also be necessary to consider neighbours in case, for example, there is a nursery room adjacent to the patient's room with only a partition wall separating the two houses. These scenarios are, however, unlikely to result in a dose of more than 0.3 mSv unless the patient has been discharged with a much higher retained activity than normally allowed. In such circumstances it would be necessary to carry out an individual risk assessment on the likely doses members of the household may receive and if appropriate, individual dose measurements for family members may be required. If an individual risk assessment has not been made and the patient insists on discharging themselves early from the hospital against the wishes of the doctor, it would be sensible to inform the appropriate authority (in the UK this is the Health Protection Agency) of the circumstances.

9.2.10 **Contingency plans**

The local rules should have contingency plans for unexpected but reasonably foreseeable adverse events such as a spill or a patient vomiting or suffering a heart attack or the evacuation of a patient in the event of a fire or electrical shutdown.

Spillage of radionuclide

If a spill occurs, staff should stay in the area and contact other staff by telephone or intercom, stating problem and asking, if necessary, that monitoring equipment is brought. Additional warning signs may be necessary to prevent entry to avoid the potential spread of contamination.

Priority should always be given to personal decontamination before proceeding with the decontamination of the area. It is important than staff only leave the area when they have been checked for contamination. If personal contamination is found help should be sought from other staff to monitor the person and identify areas of contamination. Any contaminated personal items and clothing must be removed as soon as possible and placed in a labelled polythene bag. If eyes have been contaminated they should be washed under running water immediately. Contamination on the skin should be washed with soap or suitable washing-up liquid and the skin rinsed with warm water. It is important that not too much abrasive scrubbing of the skin takes place, which could lead to the skin being broken. If contamination gets into a skin cut the area should be washed in water and bleeding encouraged. If contamination of hair occurs the hair should be washed using a wet wrung-out sponge working away from the face. The hair should then be carefully washed with shampoo and copious amounts of warm water used for rinsing. Hair should be washed in such a way that any contamination is not washed over the face or body. Hot water should not be used as it may increase skin absorption. If internal contamination is suspected physics or other appropriate staff should be contacted immediately to provide internal monitoring. All contaminated items should be placed in a suitably marked plastic bag and stored safely until the bag can be disposed through the normal route for radioactive waste or kept to decay to background levels.

Vomiting following administration

Vomiting following radionuclide administration is a possible adverse affect. Occasionally this will not be controlled by antiemetic medication. If the dose was given intravenously then the guidance given for a spill would be adequate. See Appendix 9.2 for practical details for dealing with such an episode.

Emergency care

There may be occasions when it will be necessary to deal with cardiac arrests in patients following therapy using unsealed sources. In such circumstances care of the patient must take priority over radiation protection issues. If a direct reading dosimeter is available it should be given to a member of the cardiac arrest team. Measures designed to control exposure to infection and drugs will provide adequate protection against radioactive contamination. In particular gloves and lab coats or other protective clothing should be worn, mouth to mouth resuscitation must not be undertaken and direct contact with body fluids must be avoided as far as possible. In addition to these precautions the cardiac staff should be instructed to try to work as far from the patient as they can without reducing the quality of the care they are able to give. On leaving the area the ward staff should assist the cardiac team to monitor themselves and any equipment used.

Clinical investigations

Routine investigations should be avoided until after the restriction period has passed. If it becomes necessary to take pathology samples from the patient these must be labelled with a radiation warning trefoil before being sent to the laboratory. If the laboratory is not authorized to handle radioactive samples prior advice from the RPA or must be obtained. In the event of X-ray or other investigations being required the RPA must ensure that staff are aware of the hazard and any equipment used is monitored and if necessary decontaminated following use.

9.3 **Controlling patient doses**

The IR(ME)R lays down the majority of the measures to protect patients undergoing exposures to ionizing radiations. The more practical implications of various aspects of these regulations will be detailed in the following sections.

9.3.1 **Duty holders**

The key principles of IR(ME)R are justification of the treatment and optimization of the process. Optimization should ensure all exposures of target tissues are individually planned and doses to non-target tissues are kept as low as reasonably practicable consistent with the desired radiotherapeutic outcome. For treatments using unsealed radionuclides the treatment regimen for each patient must be assessed on an individual basis. Standard activities may, however, be used where this is appropriate.

The following staff groups hold specific duties under these regulations: the employer, who must provide a framework through the provision of written procedures (referred to as the employer's procedures) and standard operating protocols; the practitioner, who has to justify and authorize each individual medical exposure; the operator, who undertakes practical aspects of the medical exposure and the referrer, who must provide sufficient relevant clinical information to enable the justification of the medical exposure. A medical physics expert (MPE) (normally a physicist appointed at principal level or above) must also be involved and available to provide advice.

Although employers might delegate the implementation of their duties under these regulations the responsibility for compliance will still remain with them. A committee, often designated as the medical exposures committee (MEC), needs to be established to oversee compliance with these regulations.

The practitioner for unsealed source treatments will normally be the Administration of Radioactive Substances Advisory Committee (ARSAC) (see Section 9.8) certificate holder for the treatments. Justification of the treatment cannot be delegated and must therefore be carried out by the practitioner. In practice this means the practitioner must sign the treatment prescription form.

In the process of justification, the practitioner must take into account; the specific objectives of the exposure and the characteristics of the individual involved; the total potential benefits; the detriment the exposure may cause; and consideration of alternative treatments not involving ionizing radiations. In practice, the first measure is to select the radiopharmaceutical that will provide the required clinical information or treatment with the least dose detriment to the patient.

The process for authorizing a procedure has been carried out as prescribed by the practitioner may be delegated, under written guidelines issued by the practitioner, to a suitably trained operator. For clinical reasons, it is most often appropriate for this to be delegated to a medical doctor who has been designated as an operator.

In some cases, the practitioner may also undertake practical aspects of an exposure, e.g. the administration of a radionuclide. In these circumstances, the practitioner acts as an operator. The functions and responsibilities of all operators and practitioners must be clearly defined within standard operating procedures.

9.3.2 Prior information to patients and patient preparation

Information must be given to the patient and consent obtained before administration. The consent process must ensure that the patient is not pregnant and if appropriate, the patient must be made aware that they will have to cease breast-feeding. At the time of giving information and obtaining consent a form of risk assessment should made to determine the patient's self-care ability.

To ensure optimum uptake of the radionuclide therapy in some cases particular drugs and or foods must be discontinued for a period of time before administration.

Some treatments can cause nausea so prior administration of an antiemetic may be required. For intravenous administration prior cannulation is helpful. Where the treatment dose is given by slow effusion the syringe pump will need to be shielded. Any patient monitoring, such as blood pressure, that is required during and/or immediately after administration should be undertaken as remotely as possible. If a patient is a child or very distressed the use of sedation should be considered.

9.3.3 Pregnancy and breast feeding

The pregnancy status for all females of reproductive capacity (normally between the ages of 12 and 55 years) must be established before any exposure to ionizing radiation begins. Pregnancy is normally a contraindication to therapies using unsealed sources. Exposure to the fetus can occur from both the external exposure from the radionuclide deposited in the mother and from placental transfer of the radionuclide. The latter exposure is of particular importance if administration has taken place once organ development has begun and can be of considerable concern for longer-lived radionuclides that reside in the mother during organogenesis.

A significant exposure to a breast-fed infant can result from radioactivity expressed in breast milk of women who have recently undergone unsealed source therapies. It is therefore essential that female patients are asked if they are breast feeding as it may be necessary to advise them to cease this activity.

9.3.4 Quality assurance and clinical evaluation

There must be a record kept of the clinical evaluation of any diagnostic or therapeutic exposure, detailing the resulting diagnostic findings or therapeutic implications. If it is known that no clinical benefit or evaluation will occur the administration is not justified and should not take place. The amount of administered activity and the delivered dose should also be included in this record. To ensure such outcomes are effective, there should be a quality management system in place and clinical audits should be routinely undertaken.

9.3.5 Practitioner and operator training

Practitioners and operators are required to be able to demonstrate that they have achieved adequate training to carry out their work as designated. The syllabus of theoretical training operators and practitioners are expected to have received is outlined in the IR(ME)R Schedule 2[5]. In addition to this aspect of theoretical training, operators and practitioners are expected to have received adequate practical training. The amount of training that would need to be covered will depend on the range of activities carried out. Practitioners will need to hold an ARSAC (see Section 9.8) certificate and normally, certificates will only be issued to consultant level medical doctors who can demonstrate adequate experience to the certificate issuing body. A nurse administering radiopharmaceuticals might be expected to receive 30–40 hours training, of which half this time would be supervised practical instruction. Up-to-date and separate records must be kept showing the date on which training was completed and the nature of the training. On-going up-to-date training must also be demonstrated after qualification. This training should include elements of radiation protection as applied to new practices, procedures, and techniques.

Practical aspects of medical exposures might be undertaken by a person training to be an operator, as long as they are under the supervision of a person already appropriately trained. This is not true for persons training to be practitioners. They must be adequately trained before being allowed to justify any treatment.

There is no duty on the referrer to be specifically trained under the regulations. However, any referrer should have the same level of competence to refer patients as that expected from a medically trained professional. The employer's procedure might therefore stipulate that the referrer must be trained to the same level of competence as that expected from doctors for specified referrals.

9.4 **Patient discharge**

The main factors that determine whether a patient may be given radiation clearance for discharge are: the radionuclide administered; the residual activity in the patient; the domestic home circumstances, and method and length of journey home. Patients should be given written advice (Appendix 9.3) regarding their conduct with other persons following discharge from hospital. This should include advice on travelling home and any future overseas travel. If overseas travel is planned they should be given documentation to carry describing the treatment given and contact details of the treating centre. It may be necessary to delay returning to work until the appropriate restriction period has passed. This is intended to help restrict doses to any persons who may be exposed through contact with the patient. Patients should also be given advice about the planning of future pregnancy. Guidance regarding the length of time between radionuclide therapy and conception is given in ARSAC (see Section 9.8) documentation[8]. In the case of children or those mentally incapacitated, instructions should be provided to the patient's carer or manager of a care home. Where children are able to understand, the instructions should be given to them also.

If a patient is to be transferred to another hospital or nursing home, information regarding the treatment administered, the retained activity and any precautions should accompany the patient. Before arranging the transfer it is necessary to check that the receiving institution is authorized to discharge the amount and type of radionuclide the patient will release into the local sewer.

Precautions may be required for post mortem and/or burial or cremation. Advice should be sought from a RPA if a patient dies soon after receiving therapy with radioactive material. The maximum residual activities of radionuclides where no special precautions for burial or cremation following death of a patient need to be taken are given in Table 9.2. Embalming should not normally be carried out if death occurs within the period covered by the instruction card above.

9.5 **Medical research**

Medical research in the UK must be approved by the Central Office Research Ethics Committee (COREC). Any uses of ionizing radiations must be identified to COREC whether or not they are part of the routine clinical requirements for the patient group or only required as part of the research study. All exposures must be justified by an IR(ME)R practitioner and a dose and risk evaluation must be provided by a suitable RPA or a suitable MPE. A dose

Table 9.2 Maximum activities of radionuclides for disposal in corpses without special precautions[6]

Radionuclide	Burial (MBq)	Cremation (MBq)
^{131}I	400[a]	400*
^{125}I seeds	4000[†]	See[§]
^{103}Pd seeds	15000*	See[§]
^{90}Y colloid	2000[†]	70[‡]
^{198}Au colloid	400*	100[‡]
^{32}P	2000[†]	30[‡]
^{89}Sr	2000[†]	200[‡]

*Based on external dose rate.

[†]Based on bresstrahlung dose at 0.5 m.

[‡]Based on contamination hazard (assuming radionuclides remain in ash).

[§]Normally to be avoided–seeds are normally sealed sources that will not be dispersed during cremation. Possibility of removal of sources to be considered with due attention and communication given
to crematorium staff and discussed with Statutory inspectors.

constraint or target dose must be identified in the application. A dose constraint establishes the maximum exposure any patient recruited into the study will be allowed to receive. Where there is a perceived benefit to the patients from the research exposures, a target dose can be set instead of a dose constraint. This is the dose that the study aims to achieve but may be exceeded if it is to the benefit of the patient involved. In studies involving multiple centres, the dose constraint needs to take into account possible variations in the standard doses delivered to patients at the different centres. For example if one centre cannot comply with the dose constraint for a diagnostic computed tomography examination required to evaluate tumour response, this centre will not be able to enter into the study unless a variation through COREC is approved. Similarly, if a lead centre uses a lower administered activity than is standard for a nuclear medicine scan, other centres will need to reduce the amount they administer for this scan unless the dose constraint has taken this into account by stipulating the standard dose rather than the lower dose. The local research ethics committee should be aware that the study can only proceed at their centre if they can comply with the dose constraint set by the lead centre.

9.6 **Exposures much greater than intended**

There is a requirement under the regulations[3,5] to inform the relevant statutory body if a patient receives a dose of ionizing radiation that was much greater than intended. If, for example, a patient was administered with 10% or more activity than intended as a result of an error that was not equipment related (e.g. human error), the DH must be immediately notified and a detailed investigation must be carried out. The DH must also be informed if a patient has received an unintended dose of radiation as a result of mistaken identification or other procedural failure. If the patient received much greater activity than intended due to an equipment fault (e.g. a faulty calibrator) the HSE must be contacted. If a patient was administered with an excess activity that did not exceed 10% the DH or HSE might still need to be contacted if, for example, a number of patients were overexposed as a result of a systems or equipment failure. In any untoward event an immediate investigation should be carried out locally to determine the effect on the patient's future clinical management or treatment and to identify the reasons for the error. Lessons can and should be learnt from episodes where it was fortuitous that the excess exposure was not significant and could have, under different circumstances, resulted in a dose that was much greater than intended. Such 'near misses' should be used to improve the processes or procedures to reduce the likelihood of similar errors occurring again.

If the patient was administered with much lower activity than intended it can have serious consequences. However, these are not notifiable, but as a matter of good practice, the employer should carry out their own investigations in such circumstances.

9.7 **Environmental issues**

Unsealed radionuclides that have been administered to a patient will have a physical decay rate dependent upon the half life of the radionuclide and a biological decay rate from the excretion that takes place. For any given radionuclide the decay rates will vary between patients depending upon retention and excretion rates (as well as varying within the patients themselves with time). In some circumstances it is important to measure the amount of activity remaining in patients (and hence deduce the amount excreted) where it is necessary to perform an accurate environmental impact hazard assessment.

9.7.1 **Regulatory environment matters**

The Radioactive Substances Act (1993)[9] requires all organizations that keep or use radioactive materials to be registered with the Environment Agency (EA). Accumulation and disposal of radioactive waste is also subject to certificates of authorization from the EA under the above Act.

Before any organization is allowed to have any radionuclide on site (there are certain exemptions—see below) they must apply to the EA specifying the radionuclides and maximum quantities they intend to use, the uses for these materials and their safe storage. A registration fee must be paid to the EA and a fee is payable for any significant variations to a registration. Records must be kept of the date and activity of receipt of any radionuclide, where it is stored, the total activity present at the end of each calendar month and the date and activity of removal from the premises. Procedures must be in place for the ordering and receipt of radioactive materials. The radiopharmaceuticals for many treatments can be purchased as a unit dose that will reduce the amount of dispensing required in the radiopharmacy. Confirmation of the correct delivery is an important aspect to consider. Staff accepting delivery should be aware of the potential serious consequences of an incorrect delivery. Measures need to be put in place for accepting out-of-hours delivery to a safe and secure location by an authorized member of staff.

A radiological hazard assessment, taking into account any critical groups (e.g. sewage workers), must be made at the application stage for an authorization to dispose of radioactive waste and the chosen routes must be justified with the organization demonstrating it has used 'best practicable means'. A fee is charged by the EA for the application and an annual subsistence charge is also payable. Records must be kept of the dates, activities, and routes of disposal and the total activities disposed in any month by each route.

In justifying the organization has achieved best practicable means of disposal, the EA will want to see alternative means of disposals considered and reasons why they have been ruled out if not used. For example, if an organization wants to discharge patient excreta containing radioiodine direct to the sewer it must be able to demonstrate that the use of abatement tanks are economically unjustifiable because the detriment to any critical group is not significant. It may, however, be necessary to have a system whereby liquid waste is delayed in its transit to the sewer. This is not usually necessary for existing installations but can be required for new installations if high activity therapies are given.

Solid radioactive waste should be stored in adequately shielded bins to reduce the external dose rate. To simplify disposal it is advisable to separate waste according to half-life. As the bins fill they should be transferred to the waste storage area. Short half-life isotopes may be stored, subject to authorization, until decayed. Longer-lived isotopes should be stored and/or disposed in accordance with the authorization. Comprehensive records of all disposals and discharges must be kept.

Institutions, such as care homes, who receive patients discharged from a hospital after undergoing treatment with unsealed sources, may be exempt under The Radioactive Substances (Hospitals) Exemption Order (1990)[10] from the need to obtain an authorization to dispose of radioactive waste.

The condition for exemption will be met if the total activity disposed to the sewer from human excreta is less than 500 MBq per month and it does not contain any α emitters. Such places do, however, need to keep records of the disposals and are also required to register with the HSE the first time they receive such a patient.

9.8 **The medicines regulations**

The Medicines (Administration of Radioactive Substances) (MARS) Regulations (1978)[11] are concerned with the protection of patients and volunteers administered with radioactive substances.

The MARS Regulations specifies that only doctors (normally at consultant level) or dentists, that hold a certificate issued by the Health Minister, or persons acting under their written directions, may administer radioactive substances to patients or volunteers. These certificates are granted by the ARSAC. Such certificates are site and practitioner specific and are issued for the range of substances and purposes specified by the applicant. Standard clinical licences are granted for 5 years and research licenses for 2 years.

The ARSAC will grant a certificate if they are satisfied that the qualifications and relevant experience of the applicant and the supporting services and scientific staff (physicists and radiopharmacists) are adequate.

The RPA must also sign to indicate that the arrangements for radiation safety are adequate.

9.9 **Movement and transport of sources**

Sources that are moved within or transported outside a hospital must be held within suitable and marked containers that will prevent their escape under reasonably foreseeable accidents that might occur during their movement or transport.

9.9.1 **Movement of sources within a hospital**

For movement of sources within a hospital it is important to consider the means of transport. For example, where a trolley is used to transport sources in a lead pot from a department to a ward, the possibility of the lead pot falling off the container should be minimized by using a trolley with sturdy wheels and maintaining a low centre of gravity where practicable.

9.9.2 **Transport of sources outside a hospital**

The transport of sources outside a hospital are governed by the Radioactive Material (Road Transport) Act 1991[12], which provides the mechanism for the provision of The Radioactive Material (Road Transport) Regulations, 2002 (SI No. 1093)[13] and The Carriage of Dangerous Goods and Use of Transportable Pressure Equipment Regulations 2004 SI No. 568[14].

The above regulations are designed to ensure a high level of safety of people, property, and the environment against exposure to radiation. The regulations have strict rules governing the type of packages that may be used for the transport, the warning signs that have to be used, the consignment details that have to be completed and the training of drivers. It is outside the scope of this book to detail these requirements and the RPA or in-house specialist should be consulted for further advice before transporting any source.

9.10 **Non-UK legislation**

Although the regulations discussed so far are specific to the UK they share a wide similarity with the regulations adopted in other member states of the European Union as they are all derived from the same European Directives. For comparison with regulations of other countries some discussion of the US legislature will be made.

The executive departments and agencies of the Federal Government of the US publishes general and permanent rules in the Federal Register, which appear as the Code of Federal Regulations (CFR). This Register is divided into 50 Titles that represent broad areas subject to Federal regulations. These Titles are then subdivided into Chapters. Each volume of the CFR is updated once each calendar year and is issued on a quarterly basis. The reader is referred to the US Government Printing Office (GPO) Titles[15] 10 (Energy), 29 (Labor), and 42 (Health). Some differences between the US (10CFR835) and UK (EU) regulations to note are:

- the annual US dose limit is 50 mSv,

- a declared (voluntary) pregnancy may be revoked in writing by the pregnant worker,

- the dose equivalent limit for the embryo/fetus from the period of conception to birth, as a result of occupational exposure of a declared pregnant worker, is 5 mSv.

The general principles serving the safe uses of radiation in the workplace are derived from the International Commission on Radiological Protection (ICRP 60, 1990 Recommendations)[16] and consequently rules and regulations governing occupational and public exposures have similar threads in Europe and the US. The regulations pertaining to patient safety can, however, significantly differ, even between European states, and these differences are outside the scope of this book to detail.

References

1. Council Directive 96/29/EURATOM (1996). *Laying down basic safety standards for the protection of the health of workers and the general public against the dangers arising from ionizing radiation.*

2. Council Directive 97/43/EURATOM (1997). *On health protection of individuals against the dangers of ionizing radiation in relation to medical exposure, and repealing Directive 84/466/Euratom.*

3. The Ionising Radiations Regulations 1999, Office of Public Sector Information (SI No. 3232).

4. HSE Books (1999). *Ionising Radiations Regulations 1999. Approved code of practice and guidance, work with ionising radiation.*

5. The Ionising Radiation (Medical Exposure) Regulations 2000, Office of Public Sector Information (SI No. 1059).

6. *Medical and Dental Guidance Notes* (2002). Institute of Physics and Engineering in Medicine.

7. Health and Safety Executive (2003). *Dose constraints for comforters and carers.* Royal Hallamshire Hospital, Research Report 155.

8. Administration of Radioactive Substances Advisory Committee (1998). *Notes for guidance on the clinical administration of radiopharmaceuticals and use of sealed radioactive sources.*

9. The Radioactive Substances Act: Elizabeth II, Chapter 12, Office of Public Sector Information, 1993.

10. The Radioactive Substances (Hospitals) Exemption Order (1990). Office of Public Sector Information (SI No. 2512).

11. Medicines (Administration of Radioactive Substances) Regulations (1978). Office of Public Sector Information (SI No. 1006).

12. Radioactive Material (Road Transport) Act (1991): Elizabeth II, Office of Public Sector Information.

13. The Radioactive Material (Road Transport) Regulations (2002). Office of Public Sector Information (SI No. 1093).

14. The Carriage of Dangerous Goods and Use of Transportable Pressure Equipment Regulations (2004). Office of Public Sector Information (SI No. 568).

15. US Government Printing Office (2005). Code of Federal Regulations, web access (2006), http://www.gpoaccess.gov/cfr/index.html.

16. ICRP Publication 60 (1991). 1990 Recommendations of the International Commission on Radiological Protection. *Annals of the ICRP* **21**(1–3).

Appendix 9.1: Information for a comforter and carer to a patient undergoing unsealed source radiotherapy

Information sheet

Your relative/friend has received (or will be receiving) a substance that remains radioactive during, and for a few days after, their treatment. This substance produces radiation in the form of gamma rays (similar to X-rays). To reduce the exposure of other people to this radiation, your relative/friend is being (or will be) treated in a specially designed room with restricted visiting times. However, it is possible for you to provide more support or care than is normally permitted if you become designated as a comforter and carer.

Implications of being a comforter and carer

There is no legal limit to the amount of radiation dose you are allowed to receive as a comforter and carer. Consequently you may receive more radiation dose than is allowed for a member of the public. It is thought that exposure to even a small amount of radiation may result in a small increased chance of developing cancer. For instance, the chance of harm resulting from the radiation dose a normal member of the public is allowed to receive is 1 in 20 000. This chance of harm is similar to:

- Smoking 40 cigarettes during a lifetime
- Driving a car for 1 year
- 9 months of normal home life.

The chance that radiation will cause harm increases with the amount of radiation dose received. We will therefore aim to limit your radiation dose to no more than five times the public radiation dose limit. This is about twice the annual radiation dose we each receive from natural sources of radiation that exist in our normal environment. It is also less than the radiation dose a member of staff is legally allowed to receive.

Providing support and care while keeping your radiation dose to the minimum

You will be provided with a digital radiation monitor. A member of staff will explain how it is used and how to record the radiation dose you receive which will be kept by us for future reference.

The following rules will help you to reduce the radiation dose you receive.

- **Time.** Spend the minimum amount of time in the same room as your relative/friend.
- **Distance.** Avoid any prolonged close contact. Keep as far away from your relative/friend as is practical.
- **Shielding.** Where possible remain behind the mobile shields within the room.

In addition, some of the radioactivity is excreted in bodily fluids such as saliva, urine, or sweat. When you are in the treatment room:

- You must wear disposable gloves and overshoes, and a gown over your own clothes.

- You must not use the en-suite toilet.

- You must not remove any article from the room.

- You must not eat or drink anything while in the room.

When leaving the treatment room, you must remove the gloves, overshoes, and gown. You will be shown where to put them. You must also wash and monitor your hands before leaving the treatment suite and you will be shown where and how to do this.

Appendix 9.2: Contingency plan agreed between medical physics expert and consultant oncologist (at Royal Marsden Hospital, Sutton)

Vomiting occurs within 30 minutes following administration of radioiodine capsule

- **Physicist:** If the capsule is visible and intact, using long handled tongs remove it to a plastic bag and place in an appropriate lead pot. Label and seal the lead container, log it as waste and store in the specimen room bunker. The patient and the treatment room can then be managed as non-active. Inform the SpR.

- **SpR:** Discharge patient when they are fit. Rebook the ablation/treatment. If the expected admission date is more than 7 days hence, prescribe thyroid hormone replacement: Liothyronine 20 µg TDS.

Vomiting occurs >30 minutes following administration of radioiodine

- **Nurse/physicist:** Follow spill procedures.

- **Physicist:** Assess the patient's whole body retention of radioiodine and inform SpR of result.

- **SpR**

  - If retention is <10% of administered activity discharge patient when they are fit. Rebook the ablation/treatment. If the expected admission date is more than 7 days hence, prescribe thyroid hormone replacement: Liothyronine 20 µg TDS.

  - If retention is <30% of administered activity discharge patient when they are fit and radiation protection restrictions allow. Rebook the ablation/treatment in approximately 3 months. Prescribe thyroid hormone replacement: Liothyronine 20 µg TDS.

- If retention is >30% of administered activity record that the treatment maybe suboptimal and ensure that a follow-up clinic appointment is made. Continue care as planned.

Appendix 9.3 Guidance notes for patients

NHS HOSPITAL TRUST:
ADDRESS:
TELEPHONE NO.:

Patient name: Hospital no:
Address: Consultant:
Details of administration: Isotope: Activity: MBq   Date:

Guidance for patients treated with radionuclides

Much of the radioactivity will be excreted from your body in urine within a day or 2 following the administration. The remainder may remain for several weeks. This in turn means that you can irradiate other people who are physically close to you.

The following simple precautions will allow the treatment to be given without causing harm to your family, friends and other persons and without undue restrictions on your daily living.

Avoid close contact with other people	for	days/until
(Try to keep at least 1 metre away)		
Sleep separately from your partner	for	days/until
(Beds should be at least 2 metres apart)		
Avoid close contact with children aged 5–16 years	for	days/until
(Try to keep hugging and holding to a minimum)		
Avoid close contact with children aged 3–5 years	for	days/until
(Try to keep hugging and holding to a minimum)		
Infants (3 years and under) should be cared for		
by someone else	for	days/until
Avoid close contact with pregnant women	for	days/until
(Try to keep at least 2 metres distance)		
You should not go to work	for	days/until
You should not go to social events, cinema,		
restaurants, etc.	for	days/until
Avoid long journeys (2 hours or more) on		
public transport	for	days/until
Avoid becoming pregnant or fathering a child	for at least	months

Other ....

I understand the restrictions explained to me by ....
Date:..............

Signature of Patient or representative ....
Date:..............

If you have any questions about your treatment or experience any unexpected problems, please contact:

....

Please carry this information with you until:...

Index

Note: Radiolabelled compounds are indexed under the name of the radioactive labels, e.g. ^{131}I-tositumomab is indexed under "I".